Longevity

Reinvent Yourself At Any Age

Maria L. Ellis, MBA

Difference Press

Washington, DC, USA

Published 2022

DISCLAIMER

Cover Design: Jennifer Stimson

Editing: Cory Hott

DISCLAIMER

ADVANCE PRAISE

"Maria Ellis's book, *Longevity,* presents a well-researched study of the importance of maintaining a healthy balance in life; whether still working or retired, it is important to strive to improve your personal habits. Eat well, exercise, participate in social activities, keep your mind active, but most of all, do something that you enjoy every day. I am reminded of a quip by several famous people, 'If I had known I was going to live so long, I would have taken better care of myself.' With people living longer, Maria's book is a great source of advice for a happier, healthier, longer life."

— Silvia D'jaen Silverman,
Past International President, Altrusa International

"I could not stop reading *Longevity: Reinvent Yourself at Any Age*! This amazing book is an excellent guide to a long productive happy life. Maria's longevity recommendations are knowledgeable, accurate, and can be followed with great ease and success. The book is well-written, understandable, and meaningful, and Maria's life is living proof that all the recommendations work."

— Nancy Mion,
Past President, American Association of University
Women New York State

"Don't buy this book! Don't read this book — *unless* you want to live an even longer, happier and healthier life. That's right; if you want that kind of life, this book is for you. Maria offers practical, realistic ideas that you can implement so quickly. In Chapter 6, she focuses on the power of humor.

There's something you can do right away: start laughing even more. If you don't think you have anything to laugh at, check in the mirror. Seriously, this is a well-written, easy-to-understand, and vitally important book if you want to live an even happier and healthier life. I'm approaching eighty-one and feel I've got a long way yet to live, thanks to the wisdom Maria is sharing on this longevity book's precious pages."

— Joel Weldon,
Hall Of Fame Professional Speaker,
Speaking Skills Coach, Genius Network Member

"Maria Ellis and I shared a passion – the quest for longevity. Independently we each decided our goal was to live well for an extreme life span. Maria has written this book; I opened a longevity center in my hometown. We chose different paths, but we are heading to the same destination. What I like and admire about this book is it is based on science, combined with love of her fellow man. She gives us a clear list of traits that will lead to a long and happy life. She guides you through an action plan to get your own life on track. Good solid information with a plan to move forward effectively. That's a good book to pick up, to read, and to share with others you care about."

— Maggie Roth,
The Longevity Center and President of
Investing Buddies

"Maria Ellis gives us in *Longevity* a commonsense blueprint on how to enjoy and have a happier lifestyle. Backed up by references to research she supports her ideas with an easy-to-follow list to do. It is a book to definitely add to your collection and to enact and have a happier, more fulfilled life."

— Michael W. Kleinman, DDS

"As a writer with family, business, and environment all being Maria's quest in life, she is best to put it in print. I consider it a privilege and a life s learning to read and understand her views on Longevity. And what makes it most gratifying is her style of writing – crisp, poignant, and revealing. I am certain it will be an enjoyable ride on *Longevity*!"

— Gunatheesan Navasivayam, MD

CONTENTS

DEDICATION

I would like to dedicate this book to my family,
Stephen, Michael, Dominique, Thomas, Kathryn,
and Maven Rose, with the hope that it will add healthy
years, even decades, to the lives of those who read this
book and create healthy lifespan habits.

FOREWORD

Maria Ellis has written her fourth book, *Longevity: Reinvent Yourself at Any Age*. Her book is about a topic that is always important, generation after generation: how to live a healthy, happy, and long life. Maria spent her entire career in the financial world, rising up the ladder at a large and prestigious bank conducting international business and now advising on wellness, freedom and legacy to business owners and high net worth individuals. Maria is also a Chopra Certified Health Instructor, and she deeply understands ayervedic wellness that addresses the whole person – physically, mentally, emotionally, and spiritually. In this process, a person's state of body, mind, and spirit are assessed and from there we journey on the road to your optimal wellness.

Maria authentically shares her knowledge and expertise in this highly readable book. She captures both the mind and the heart of the longevity process and does so in a fluid and accessible manner. Her poignant examples and stories lend further credence to the practical tips and tools that are relevant across cultures. She effortlessly captures the unique and sometimes difficult-to-articulate aspects of a well-lived life dynamic.

Maria's life story is truly inspiring. Immigrating to the United States with her family after graduating from high school in Guayaquil, Ecuador where she was born and spent her formative years, Maria pursued her BBA and MBA at the University of Massachusetts, and later enrolled in the Harvard Business School Owner-President Management program. This education allowed Maria to pursue her professional dreams and serves as a great example of the pillars in successful personal and financial wellness. Maria's analysis goes beyond simple longevity planning. She shares in detail the many aspects of longevity and wellness with ease. This is not simply a to-do list, but a holistic, strategic approach to extend your lifetime horizon and family continuity.

This book builds on the foundational tools of Maria's best-seller book, *Redefining Entrepreneurial Success: A Guide to a Healthy and Holistic Lifestyle*, which serves as a helpful reference guide as you reach each of your personal wellness and financial milestones. I should add that Maria possesses a great work ethic; she commits to doing her best in all that she takes on. In addition to her advisory services, Maria is a pro-bono consultant with the Harvard Business School Club of New York's Community Partners, whose mission is to create constructive partnerships between Harvard Business School alumni and nonprofit organizations in the greater New York City metropolitan area that seek assistance with business and management issues.

I'm proud to be a recognized leader in the field of health coaching. In 2015, I founded the Functional Medicine Coaching Academy (FMCA), a collaboration with the Institute for Functional Medicine. The curriculum offers an innovative coaching model blending functional medicine principles with positive psychology and mind-body medicine. FMCA is online and experiential, serves a global population and is fully approved by the National Board for Health and Wellness Coaching. I train people to become functional medicine health coaches and help practitioners and businesses hire them because I believe that health coaches as behavior change specialists are the key to combatting chronic disease and reducing healthcare costs.

I founded FMCA and became CEO at the age of sixty-five. An educator and licensed clinical psychologist for more than forty years, I was not about to enter retirement like so many of my contemporaries. Instead, I chose to embark on a mission-driven career. I'm passionate about my life purpose: training thousands of health coaches so that there will be a coach in every medical practice.

Like Maria, I'm a member of the Genius Network. I wrote several books, including *How to Become a Health Coach: The Career that Can Bring People Joy*, *Functional Medicine Coaching*, and *Stop Panic Attacks in 10 Easy Steps*. I'm a contributor to Forbes and a frequent podcast guest.

As you can well imagine, longevity and wellness are tremendously important to me, indeed critically important to me. If you want to know how to reinvent yourself at any age and do not know where to start, or if you need more clarity about important longevity questions, as applied to your life, Maria's book will be an invaluable font of information for all your queries. She makes this complex journey simple, clear, and fun.

—Sandra Scheinbaum, PhD

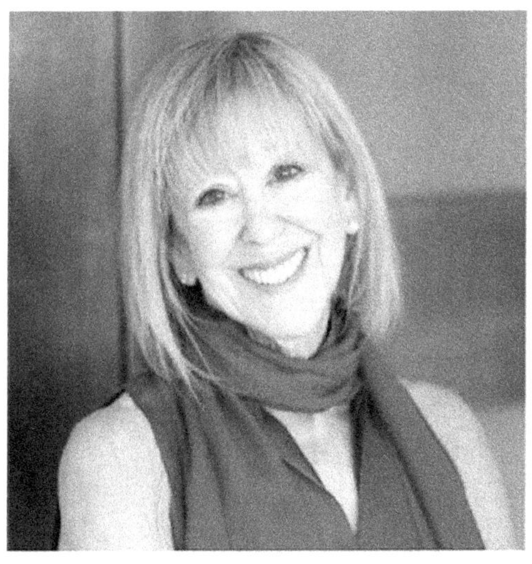

INTRODUCTION

I have known Maria Ellis for more than fifteen years as a friend and one who actively participates in high-level intellectual group discussions involving an array of worldly issues. Maria has wealth of knowledge in several fields. She is an intellectual and very loving, caring, humorous – and yet still one of us. Through Maria Ellis's counseling, writing, and teaching, she has won the admiration and hearts of many. As a Deepak Chopra's Health Certified Instructor, the driving force in Maria to write *Longevity: Reinvent Yourself at Any Age* is due to her passion to uplift the lives of everyone around – far and beyond!

Longevity, based on Chopra's Well-Being Assessment, is well written and easy to read, and is made interesting with quotes from several legends of past and present and real-life stories. It provides complete information how to get to know your real self; how to live and enjoy life to the fullest by identifying and bringing out the hidden, dormant, or suppressed strengths; how to give an expression to those strengths; the importance of self-love; how to harvest and harness energy from community and nature; the importance of give and take; how to put the clock back on your life; and more.

Longevity provides guidelines and valuable tools explaining the whys and hows for planning for the present and future; it cautions the booby traps for a comfortable, day-to-day joyous living; it teaches medical, nonmedical, self, social and legal aspects that one ought to know. And finally, it teaches choices one can and needs to make, leaving no stone unturned. The book is comprehensive and well-organized, including statistics and a complete list of places for healthy and happy living, which are well researched and laid out with common-sense advice. Although the book appears to be for the middle aged and those in their golden years, this is an encyclopedia encompassing information for the young, a guide to professionals – both medical and nonmedical – addressing several aspects for a worthy human life.

As a retired physician with knowledge in my own sphere, I had to gather the nonmedical information related to healthy living and the legal aspects through several sources. Now I have all needed information packaged within *Longevity: Reinvent Yourself at Any Age*. I not only enjoyed reading the book, but this is also the best and most user-friendly book that will find a spot on my bookshelf!

Sharada Jayagopal, MD,
East Williston, New York

1

WHY I AM NOT LIVING A HEALTHY AND HAPPY LIFE IN MY GOLDEN YEARS?

"For even if the allotted space of life be short, it is long enough in which to live honorably and well."
— Cicero

Eleanor is a married woman – sixty-five years old and living in Chicago. She has raised three children and has worked as a bookkeeper most of her life. She has two sons, thirty and thirty-five years old, and one daughter, who is twenty-nine years old. All three of her adult children have moved out of the Chicago area to pursue their career goals. Eleanor is concerned about dying young since her mother passed away at sixty-five years old from a heart condition. Eleanor, like her mother, also suffers from a heart condition, type 2 diabetes, and high blood pressure. Eleanor has two sisters, two brothers, and a few nieces and nephews who communicate only during the holidays. Eleanor has been working for a long time as a bookkeeper. She feels that there is no opportunity for advancement, and she knows that her employer can hire a younger and more qualified college graduate even at a lower salary. Eleanor feels unloved, excluded, helpless, overlooked, disenfranchised, alienated, silenced, and worthless.

Eleanor, like most of us, is looking for love in all the

wrong places. Eleanor has been married two times; her first marriage lasted seven years. She divorced her first husband after she realized that she could not change her husband's personality and lack of ambition. She wanted to raise a family, so after being divorced for four years, she married again. She made sure that her second husband would be interested in creating a prosperous and successful family. Her second husband's motto was that power isn't everything, it is the only thing.

Carl Jung identified twelve primary types that represent the range of basic human motivations (the ruler, creator/artist, sage, innocent, explorer, rebel, hero, wizard, jester, everyman, lover, and the caregiver). Each of us tends to have one dominant archetype that dominates our personality. Eleanor likes to connect with others and loves intimacy. Eleanor's talents include passion, gratitude, appreciation, and commitment, and her weakness includes her need to please others at risk of losing her identity. Her second husband likes to provide structure to the world and seeks control. His talents include responsibility and leadership, and his weakness is being authoritarian and unable to delegate. According to Carl Jung, "Where love rules, there is no will power, and where power predominates, love is lacking."

Eleanor is an example of how the lack of self-love can negatively impact you. Recognizing and practicing self-love is important because it affects every aspect of our lives. The way we feel about ourselves impacts our relationships, our careers, how much money we make, how happy we truly are, and how people perceive us. Feeling good about yourself is key to having a good life. Self-love enables you to hold yourself in high esteem and have confidence in your worth, no matter what happens around you. Your self-love will increase if you see who you are rather than seeing yourself through all the false beliefs and distortions.

Self-love starts with self-compassion, trusting others, coping with your emotions, communicating effectively, honoring your potential, and feeling authentic and confident. With self-love, just as with Eleanor, in this book you will find ways to extend your time horizon by living a healthy and happy life. As adults, you need to take responsibility for knowing your authentic or truest selves. The essence of who you are is a deep reservoir for your capacity to love and experience joy and compassion. A study at the University of Louisville, led by Michael Steger, aimed to find out if pleasure-seeking behaviors or doing good made people happier. They concluded, "The more people participated in meaningful activities, the happier they were and the more purposeful their lives felt. Pleasure-seeking behaviors, on the other hand, did not make people happier."

Many of the issues that people struggle with, such as depression, anxiety, and relationship issues, are symptoms of a lack of self-love and disconnection from their true authentic self. When people feel insecure, they can worry, feel sad, or even lash out. In contrast, when you feel confident and embrace the real you, those bad feelings are less likely to arise. In Eleanor's case, she needs to reflect on what is important to her now and reevaluate her life goals accordingly. Eleanor needs to create a one- to three-year plan with specific goals and objectives to have clarity of mind to enable her to identify the new priorities in her life. You may be experiencing the same issues as Eleanor, but that is okay, because a solution exists for you.

2

HOW I EXTENDED MY TIME HORIZON FOR ANOTHER FORTY YEARS

"There is a fountain of youth: it is your mind, your talents, the creativity you bring to your life and the lives of people you love. When you learn to tap this source, you will truly have defeated age."
— Sophia Loren

I decided to extend my life because I want to share with my family and with the world the importance of giving and for being an instrument of God's love. It has taken over seventy years to realize that it is in giving that we receive. I hope that my story will inspire you to extend the years of your life to fulfill your dreams.

I was raised in a Catholic family in Guayaquil, Ecuador. I was one of five children, and my parents work hard to provide for the family. I was raised in a happy family and always felt loved and encouraged by my parents especially my mother, Jenny, who always made me feel confident. She was the wind beneath my wings; whenever I doubted my capabilities, my mother made me feel confident that I could accomplish whatever task was in front of me on any given day. That is how I became a bilingual tour guide at sixteen years old while, at the same time, finishing high school. I worked with an international cruise line that organized international tours and brought many American tourists to

Ecuador to learn about Ecuador's flora and fauna. It was a great way to practice my English, learn about the United States, and earn some money to help pay for my extracurricular school activities, such as learning English and singing in my school choir.

After graduating from high school, it was time to leave Ecuador, my beloved country, and move to the United States to go to college and seek a brighter future. After attending UMass in Amherst, I started a career in banking, got married, and was blessed with two wonderful sons, Michael and Tommy. In addition to my banking work, I started my non-profit work. And at age twenty-eight, I was elected to be the president of the Latin American Chamber of Commerce helping business owners with the import and export businesses. I became a vice president at Citibank at thirty-four, and my successful banking career brought me to Chicago, Los Angeles, and finally to New York City. It was a rewarding time in my life, and I was living the dream. It was while working in New York City in 1987 when I fell in love with the mission of the American Association of University Women to promote pay equity and education for women and girls. I find it rewarding to help women and girls pursue their college dreams, graduate, and obtain gainful employment serving others and the community. I will share with you three of the many successful stories. These three special women friends – Jessica, Ayesha, and Paola – received fellowships from the American Association of University Women that enabled them to complete their college education and become an asset to their respective communities.

Jessica completed her doctorate in philosophy at Stony Brook University this past December and was the recipient of AAUW's American Dissertation Fellowship for the 2016–2017 school year. Her research focuses on psychological torture – also known as non-state torture – and its long-term effects on human consciousness. The practical example that she uses in her work is a type of domestic violence known as "coercive control." She aims to explain why many women who suffer from this abuse often refuse to leave an abusive partner even when given the clear opportunity to do so. She concludes that the abuser's combined use of aggression and affection causes a form of anxiety in the victim that causes her to become addicted to him. This ultimately means that she will require rehabilitation to "get clean" just like any other recovering addict. Jessica has transitioned from academia to nonprofit outreach to use her research to aid those suffering from this affliction. Through her research on psychological torture, Jessica is able to raise awareness to help others in her community and become an instrument of God's love. Best of all, her sense of purpose is linked to a longer, healthier, more satisfying life.

Ayesha is an Emmy-winning digital media native working in the intersection of technology and media. She is currently a coordinator with PRO Unlimited at the News Partnerships team at Facebook. Her career began in Singapore, where she studied information engineering and media at Nanyang Technological University. She moved back to her hometown in Kathmandu, Nepal, and joined *Nepali Times* as the online producer. I first met Ayesha Shakya when she was an International Fellow with the American Association of University Women. The AAUW International Fellowship provides support for women pursuing full-time graduate or postdoctoral study in the United States to women who are not U.S. citizens or permanent residents. Ayesha was pursuing a master's degree at New York University at the time of her fellowship. Her commitment to promote education for girls and women has carried on to her current position at Malala Fund, an international, non-profit organization that advocates for girls' education. She currently serves in a critical leading role at Malala Fund, cultivating the leading non-profit research organization's successful digital strategy and creating innovative digital content that has greatly impacted the organization's reach and success in its mission. Through her digital work, Ayesha raises awareness and promote education for girls, giving her a purposeful, happy life that increases her longevity.

Paola is fully committed to the development of sustainable communities and to the empowerment of women. She worked in Colombia and New York improving housing conditions, generating new housing units, and creating jobs and social services for low-income communities. Paola was involved in the development of more than 300 affordable housing units in New York with on-site social services for its residents and in the improvements of more than 15,000 housing units in Colombia through a micro-credit model for low-income communities. She managed a job creation and social services program (including education and empowerment toolkits, and services to eradicate all forms of violence against women) for women heads of households in Colombia, generating more than 300 jobs per year. Paola had the opportunity to study abroad in Kenya, Brazil, and Turkey to learn about grassroots organizations and urban planning strategies at the local level. Paola's commitment to improve housing conditions, generating new housing units, and creating jobs and social services for low-income communities gives her meaning and purpose to her life and increases her life span.

Like Sophia Loren, I also believe that there is a fountain of youth. It is our minds, our talents, the creativity we bring to our lives, and the lives of the people we love. When we learn to tap into this source, we will truly defeat age. I have always been goal driven, and I have lived my life in alignment with the following twelve life categories in my life vision. You, too, have the choice to imagine your own future and then design your life around your vision. Create your own life vision. What would give you purpose, happiness, and longevity? Take time to reflect and create the grandest vision for your life.

1. HEALTH AND FITNESS

You must define exactly what you want, why you want it, and what you need to do to get it. While it is impossible to avoid all stress in life, minimizing stressors and managing the way you respond to stress can have important benefits. A healthy lifestyle includes stress management as well as a nutritional diet and regular activity.

2. INTELLECTUAL

Intellectual wellness is the ability to be open to new ideas, critical thinking, and learning new skills to create the potential for sharing with others and use it for betterment of the community. Intellectual wellness promotes creative mental stimulation as well as learning new and exciting things. A good way to increase your intellectual wellness is to read for fun.

3. EMOTIONAL

It is important to explore the nature of your emotions and discover how you can further develop your emotional intelligence. Make your emotions work for you, instead of living in reaction mode. Emotional intelligence refers to our ability to understand and effectively use our different emotions. Emotional intelligence is linked to better mental and physical health and overall life satisfaction.

4. CHARACTER

This is the foundational category that affects every other area of your life. You will define the person you need to become in order to achieve the life you desire. You'll learn how to consciously choose the character traits you want to build into your life and develop a strategy for accomplishing them.

5. SPIRITUAL

Everyday life is impossible without holding your own set of beliefs. Most people are guided by a belief in the work they do, their religion, loyalty to their family, and all kinds of values they hold dear.

6. LOVE RELATIONSHIPS

You'll achieve clarity on what you want in this area of your life and identify what steps you can take to create and nurture an extraordinary love relationship. What would your ideal love relationship look like? Is trust one of the most important factors in a relationship? How about communication? Communication is key in any relationship to define boundaries.

7. PARENTING

This is a profound exploration for parents. This category is important because the future of the whole human race depends on at least some of us doing it right. You will have to decide what kind of parent you want to be. According to psychologists who study parenting, there are four main styles of parenting: autocratic, authoritative, permissive, and unengaged. The styles differ in terms of how much involvement you have in your child's life and how much control you try to exert over your child's behavior.

8. SOCIAL

Here, you'll thoughtfully evaluate your relationships with friends and extended family. You'll come to understand which relationships contribute positively to your life and which ones drain you. You'll learn what actions you can take to strengthen your most important relationships and what you can do to let unhealthy relationships go.

9. CAREER

Explore the meaning and rewards of a great career. Learn strategies to take any career to a higher level and make more money in the process. Proactivity is required for career success. First, it's a mindset. You need to realize that no one cares more about your career and its financial impact than you do. You need to be proactive if you want career advancement.

10. FINANCIAL

This is an important category, and you need to deeply explore the true nature of money —what it means to you, what it is, where it comes from, and how wealth is created and achieved. This process of self-discovery, will enable you to create a financial plan to achieve financial freedom, leading you to a better quality of life based on your life vision.

11. QUALITY OF LIFE

This category you will identify how you wish to spend the hours, the days, and the years of your life. You will discover how it can lead to rewarding spiritual, intellectual, and emotional breakthroughs and improve who you are as a human being. Quality of life is an overarching term for the quality of the various domains in human life.

12. LIFE VISION

You have thought through your entire life, one category at a time. Now, you're going to experience the life you intend to create. For instance, if you're facing a financial challenge, you might sometimes find that the solution lies not in focusing directly on money or your career but on your intellectual life or even your life vision. If you have a vision for your life, you'll always know what areas of life to focus on at any given time, and how to create extraordinary success in each of them without sacrifice or compromise.

All these categories are important for a happy life, yet you will find out that some categories become more important at different times in your life cycle. For instance, when I made a goal to extend my life for another forty years, my health and financial wellness categories became a higher priority. Being a financial advisor myself, it was important not only to have a healthy longevity but also to have the financial means to continue to maintain my comfortable and happy lifestyle. Therefore, I created a yearly budget based on my lifetime goals that shows me how much money I could spend on an annual basis without depleting my retirement fund. If you are exploring the idea of extending your lifespan, you also must be vigilant of both your health and your financial wellbeing.

All of these twelve categories work together when creating your grandest vision. For example, when it comes to how to improve your health and fitness, your intellectual life holds the power to move you quickly and forcefully toward your life's goals. In closing, keep in mind, Carl Yung's wise words, "Your vision will become clear only when you can look into your heart. Who looks outside, dreams; who looks inside, awakes." Also, keep the words of late mythologist Joseph Campbell in mind and "follow your bliss."

3

A BLUEPRINT TO A HEALTHIER, HAPPIER, AND LONGER LIFE

"Discipline is the bridge between goals and accomplishments."
— Jim Rohn

Do you dream of adding years to your life to enable you to see your grandchildren grow but have no idea where to start or how to achieve this longevity goal? Well, throughout this book, I will share the steps that you will take to move from feelings of despair to having the skills, tools, and resources to live a healthier, happier, and longer life.

In Chapter 4, you are going to learn about the importance of including laughter and music in your life. Laughter is a potent releaser of endorphins (the chemicals that help us to feel good). Laughing with friends releases endorphins in our brains via opioid receptors. Music and laughter can also bring lasting benefits to your state of mind and how therapeutic music has been clinically proven to improve sleep, relieve stress, and gain more energy for your day.

In Chapter 5, I will teach you about the science of fasting and longevity, a fasting-mimicking diet, and the Mediterranean diet.

In Chapter 6, I will teach you the importance of demography and diversity. What does demographics have to do with longevity, including showing you how the place you live, and your environment have an important role in your longevity?

In Chapter 7, I will show you how clean air matters for a healthy lifestyle and the risk of air pollution and Alzheimer's risk.

In Chapter 8, I will teach you about interventions to reduce aging, including how longevity must begin in early life, and the importance of your immune system and healthy brain. I will also teach you ways to naturally relieve stress and anxiety, and I will show you how volunteering and developing friends to find significance.

In Chapter 9, I will share relevant information about caregivers, including elder abuse, care managers, and families providing the right support.

Chapter 10 is a bonus chapter in which I will inform you about new technologies, advanced research, and digital health solutions, including powerful tools to increase health care quality and access. I will also show you the biology of aging versus chronological age and the dissemination of information about effective public health measures to support healthy longevity.

In Chapter 11, I will remind you of the reasons why you are unlikely to take action and what is likely to happen if you don't.

Chapter 12 is my desire for you to live a healthier and longer life. I will recap and clarify the importance of having a blueprint to live healthier and longer.

But how would you know that you are living your life to the fullest? How about taking a quick survey of your current lifestyle? As a Chopra Certified Health Instructor, I am encouraging you to reflect and journal on the following Chopra Well-Being Assessment. It will serve you as a guide in self-reflection to recognize the areas of your life that you are inspired to focus on while letting go of those that are not a priority. It's about aligning with your life rather than going against your flow.

Think of this assessment as a magnifying glass into your life. Focus on what you need and delete what is no longer serving you. If something isn't a priority, reflect on why that is. Instead of assuming you're not motivated, perhaps recognize that there's a barrier or unrealistic expectation you're placing on yourself unnecessarily. This isn't a checklist of things you should or shouldn't be doing. It's a check-in to evaluate what is right for you. Use this journaling to help you reveal realistic, true, heartfelt intentions for you, as you are. Once you have finished journaling, save it so you can look back and reflect on your life journey.

CHOPRA WELL-BEING ASSESSMENT

1. What are the three most important areas you would like to put more energy toward in your life? List a few actions you will take to accomplish this. For example, writing and publishing, on a timely basis, this longevity book for you filled my heart with great joy.
2. Describe the time or times you feel the most inspired and accomplished – the most you. What are you doing? Who are you with? How do you feel in those moments? For example, in my case, one of the times that I feel the most inspired and accomplished is when I am mentoring the College of Mount Saint Vincent or the New York Institute of Technology graduating students, advocating pay equity, and promoting education for women and girls.
3. What are some ways you can avoid burnout in these areas? For example, turning off work notifications after hours or taking a rest day from intense physical exercises.
4. Are there any areas that aren't a priority for you right now? If it's something within your control, how can you put energy toward it? If it's not, how will you practice acceptance in this area? For example, it has been in my mind to obtain a PhD, but I have not yet put energy toward it. I need to decide

whether obtaining a PhD is important enough for me right now or is a longer-term goal.

After completing this survey, one of my clients, Julie, was able to free herself from a life of boredom, disappointments, and pill overdoses. She was able to focus on what she needed and eliminated what was no longer serving her. She started journaling every day, and she created a vision for herself. Journaling helped Julie to clarify her intentions, and she created a strategy to implement her new life vision. After making hard decisions, such as divorcing her husband, she became fully engaged in an enjoyable career, focusing in raising her daughter and tending to her educational needs.

If you are experiencing similar issues and/ or are not happy with your life, ask what the most important areas of your life right now that need to be changed are. What do you need to do change in your attitude or behavior to start living well again? How can you create a new vision for your life? Who can help you achieve your goals? Ask for professional help as needed. It is your life that is at peril.

In your journey to wellbeing, one of the most important practices is accepting and loving yourself just as you are. Proceed with compassion and awareness, and make a list of three reasons you are proud of yourself. Once you make your list, turn them into positive affirmations, beginning each affirmation with "I am…" Say them to yourself every morning, mean and believe them. Some of my daily affirmations are, "I am love, I am beautiful, I am abundance, I am optimistic, I am compassionate," et cetera.

In conclusion, I encourage you to start and/ or continue to reflect and affirm your good habits to live a healthier, happier, and longer life. For instance, your daily affirmations could include a healthy mind and body; satisfactory work; fun, creativity, and play; life purpose, resilience; abundance; environment; nature; connection; relationships; and self-love. Support a restful, alert mind through mindful awareness for calmer and contentment. Incorporate healthy habits into my routine to support a joyful, energetic body.

Work to uncover your true self and access higher states of consciousness for lightness of being. Cultivate focus, inspiration, and compassion, and enjoy work that is meaningful to you. Make time for play and creativity by recognizing what makes you come alive. Find inspiration in daily life. Follow the path to your *dharma*, or life's purpose, and discover lifelong passion and alignment in everything you do. Navigate life's beauty and challenges with self-care tools to build self-regulation and adaptability. Cultivate abundance, trusting in the infinite organizing power of the universe to meet your needs. Be intentional in connecting with nature to stay grounded and centered. Strive to deepen your relationship with yourself and others to form meaningful connections and build community. And use self-care practices to cultivate your self-love and gracefully accept every facet of your being.

4

DEMOGRAPHY, DIVERSITY, AND LIFESPAN

"Life expectancy in America is about seventy-nine, we should be able to live to ninety-two. Somewhere along the line, we're leaving thirteen years on the table. So my quest is — how do we g et those extra thirteen years? And how do we make those extra thirteen years good years?"

— Dan Buettner

According to census demographics data in 2021, 331.9 million people lived in the United States. The population grew by 392,665 from 2020 to 2021, or 0.1 percent, the lowest annual growth rate since the nation's founding. In the United States, the population is changing and growing more diverse. Immigration made up 62.3 percent of annual growth as births decreased and deaths increased.

2021 US POPULATION BY RACE AND ETHNICITY

- White: 60.1 percent
- Black: 12.2 percent
- Hispanic: 18.5 percent
- Asian: 5.6 percent
- American Indian/ Alaska Native: 0.7 percent
- Native Hawaiian/ Other Pacific Islander: 0.2 percent

- Multiple Races: 8 percent

The non-Hispanic white population fell below 60 percent in the 2020 census, with Hispanic Americans accounting for 51 percent of population growth between 2010 and 2020. The median age for Hispanic Americans is 29.8, nearly nine years lower than the median age of 38.5 for the entire US population. About 8 percent of the Hispanic population is over 65, compared to 17 percent of the total population. 31 percent of Hispanic Americans are under eighteen, compared to 22 percent of the nation.

Nearly one out of every 715 people in the US died from coronavirus in 2021. That's 464,000 people. In 2021, 34 million Americans tested positive for COVID-19, up 70 percent from 20 million in 2020. As of January 31, 2022, 75 percent of the population had received at least one COVID-19 vaccine. Twenty-seven percent had received a booster shot. Personal healthcare spending was $3.4 trillion in 2020, a 4.5 percent increase from 2019. Twenty-eight million Americans (8.6 percent of the population) did not have health insurance in 2020, up from 8 percent in 2019. Preliminary data shows that 3.4 million people died in 2021, 13 percent more than in 2019. The top three causes – heart disease, cancer, and COVID-19 – accounted for 50 percent of deaths. The federal government spent $141 billion on public health in 2021 – a 21 percent decrease from 2020, but more than double its 2019 public health spending.

The population is getting older, and more people are living alone. Starting in 2030, when all boomers will be older than sixty-five, older Americans will make up 21 percent of the population, up from 15 percent today. By 2060, nearly one in four Americans will be sixty-five years and older, the number of eighty-five-plus will triple, and the country will add a half-million centenarians. Based on available demographic evidence, the human lifespan shows no sign of approaching a fixed limit imposed by biology or other factors. Rather, both the average and the maximum human life span have increased steadily overtime for more than a century.

Each day, our society becomes more and more diverse. You meet more people daily, and each one brings a new perspective about something into your lives. People everywhere have different opinions and ideas that we might never have thought of. Your lives are filled with people, each with different backgrounds and experiences, whom we interact with every day. Diversity shows itself peeking out from the corner in many ways, including race, sexuality, culture, values, religion, gender, and an abundance of other ways. Diversity has not always been welcomed with open arms, but more and more, we see people opening their minds to others' ideas.

Embracing diversity into your life is how you find all the brilliant ideas out there in the world. It is how you learn more about the world around us. By exploring other ideas, beliefs, and lifestyles with an open mind, you open yourself to exercise creativity and problem solving by looking at things from other lenses. If you only take one perspective about events in the world, you will never understand the other perspectives behind them and, therefore, lock yourself into a sort of closed-minded ideology that has only led to prejudice throughout history. Diversity brings beauty and strength to your life.

I will now share with you one of my favorite poems by Maya Angelou, who personifies diversity, beauty, and strength.

> *Pretty women wonder where my secret lies.*
> *I'm not cute or built to suit a fashion model's size*
> *But when I start to tell them,*
> *They think I'm telling lies.*
> *I say, It's in the reach of my arms*
> *The span of my hips,*
> *The stride of my step,*
> *The curl of my lips.*
> *I'm a woman*
> *Phenomenally.*

MARIA L. ELLIS

Phenomenal woman,
That's me.

I walk into a room
Just as cool as you please,
And to a man,
The fellows stand or
Fall down on their knees.
Then they swarm around me,
A hive of honeybees.
I say, It's the fire in my eyes,
And the flash of my teeth,
The swing in my waist,
And the joy in my feet.
I'm a woman Phenomenally.
Phenomenal woman,
That's me.

Men themselves have wondered
What they see in me.
They try so much
But they can't touch
My inner mystery.
When I try to show them
They say they still can't see.
I say, It's in the arch of my back,
The sun of my smile,
The ride of my breasts,
The grace of my style.
I'm a woman Phenomenally.
Phenomenal woman,
That's me.

Now you understand
Just why my head's not bowed.
I don't shout or jump about
Or have to talk real loud.

When you see me passing
It ought to make you proud.
I say, It's in the click of my heels,
The bend of my hair,
the palm of my hand,
The need of my care,
'Cause I'm a woman Phenomenally.
Phenomenal woman,
That's me.

Phenomenal Woman, Maya Angelou

Does the place you live and your environment have an important role in your longevity? Living a long and happy life depends largely on your lifestyle choices. Everything from what you eat to how much you exercise to the speed at which you walk affects your lifespan in major ways. But according to an extraordinary new assessment by the US Burden of Disease Collaborators, where you live also matters. According to an article written by Diana Bruk and published in BestLife, a recent study analyzed 333 causes and eighty-four risk factors of mortality from 1990 to 2016 to provide the first-ever assessment of patterns of health in America state by state. The highest life expectancy went to Hawaii, which clocked in at 81.3 years. The lowest went to Mississippi, where the life expectancy was only 74.7 years. The life expectancy of every state was assessed to inform national health priorities for research, clinical care, and policy. But they are also useful to keep in mind, especially if you're either retired or self-employed and therefore have the freedom to live anywhere you want. The following are some of the states that have some of the highest life expectancies.

Hawaiians make it to the ripe old age of 81.3. But you don't have to live on a beach on one of the smaller islands to enjoy its benefits. After all, Honolulu recently ranked as number one in waste removal, air pollution, infectious diseases, and water quality in a study on the best places to live abroad.

California is the closest in America that you can get to Sardinia, where people regularly live over the age of ninety. With an average life expectancy of 80.9 years, Californians aren't too far behind, though, probably because they follow the same rules for longevity. Sardinia's five secrets to longevity are eat a lean, plant-based diet accented with meat, drink goat's milk, put family first, participate in daily physical activity, and drink a glass of red wine daily.

Connecticut, where the life expectancy is 80.8 years, is one the richest state in America, and wealthy people do tend to live longer. But as Warren Buffet recently warned people, it's important to remember that money does not equal happiness. Research has identified positivity as one of the personality traits that are guaranteed to extend your life.

Minnesotans are a cheerful bunch, which is probably part of what makes their average life expectancy 80.8 years.

The Affordable Care Act was modeled after Massachusetts's universal healthcare. Access to good healthcare is one of the deciding factors of longevity, which is why Massachusetts clocks in at 80.4 years.

Washington, where the average life expectancy is 80.2 years, is consistently ranked as one of the most environmentally friendly states in America. It's also got three national parks within state boundaries for people who love to hike. And research has shown that it is possible to walk your way to a longer life.

I know that the place where you live and your environment have an important role in your longevity. Living a long and happy life depends largely on your lifestyle choices. Everything from what you eat to how much you exercise to the speed at which you walk affects your lifespan in major ways. One of my clients, Thomas, decided to move his family from crowded New York City during the 2020 COVID-19 pandemic to a small town in upstate New York. Thomas enjoys the outdoors, and both he and his wife can work from home. Of course, they miss the diversity that New York City offers, but the country lifestyle, hiking, and clean air suit them best.

According to the *New York Times* bestselling author Dan Buettner, the top happiest cities in the United States are, in order,

1. Boulder, Colorado
2. Santa Cruz and Watsonville, California
3. Charlottesville, Virginia
4. Fort Collins, Colorado
5. San Luis Obispo, Paso Robles, and Arroyo Grande, California
6. San Jose, Sunnyvale, and Santa Clara, California
7. Provo and Orem, Utah
8. Bridgeport and Stamford, Connecticut
9. Barnstable, Massachusetts
10. Anchorage, Alaska
11. Naples, Immokalee, and Marco Island, Florida
12. Santa Maria and Santa Barbara, California
13. Salinas, California
14. North Port, Sarasota, and Bradenton, Florida
15. Honolulu, Hawaii
16. Ann Arbor, Michigan
17. San Francisco, Oakland, and Hayward, California
18. Colorado Springs, Colorado
19. Manchester and Nashua, New Hampshire
20. Oxnard, Thousand Oaks, and Ventura, California
21. Washington D.C., Arlington, and Alexandria, Virginia
22. Minneapolis and St. Paul, Minnesota
23. San Diego and Carlsbad, California
24. Portland and South Portland, Maine

With lifespans growing ever longer, the opportunities for our third stage of life have never been greater. In a recent summit on aging, Maria Shriver interviewed Dan Buettner, explorer, journalist, National Geographic Fellow, and *New York Times* bestselling author; and Dr. Laura L. Carstensen, professor of psychology and public policy at Stanford

University and founding director of the Stanford Center on Longevity. They talked about why our world must undergo a massive shift in consciousness to better support our increasing longevity and what we can learn from cultures that are living the longest, healthiest lives.

Dr. Laura L. Carstensen believes that age-integrated cities, workplaces, and households are good for our health and changes in behavior toward older people can lead to a positive shift in attitudes. Also, Dr. Carstensen talked about the need to create new language and vocabulary for aging and the need for policy changes that might create more sustainable environments for aging.

Dan Buettner talked about the places in the world – dubbed Blue Zones – where people live the longest, healthiest lives. Dan now works in partnership with governments, large employers, and other entities to apply lessons learned from the Blue Zones to improve lives and communities. He is the author of the new book *The Blue Zones Challenge: A 4-Week Plan for a Longer, Better Life.*

What began as a National Geographic expedition led by Dan Buettner to uncover the secrets of longevity evolved into the discovery of the five places around the world where people consistently live over 100 years old, dubbed the Blue Zones. Dan and his team of demographers, scientist and anthropologists were able to distill the evidence-based common denominators of these Blue Zones into nine commonalities listed below that they call the Power Nine. They have since taken these principles into communities across the United States working with policy makers, local businesses, schools, and individuals to shape the environments of the Blue Zones Project Communities. What has been found is that putting the responsibility of curating a healthy environment on an individual does not work, but through policy and environmental changes, the Blue Zones Project Communities have been able to increase life expectancy, reduce obesity, and make the healthy choice the easy choice for millions of Americans.

A Danish Twin Study established that only about 20 percent of how long the average person lives is dictated by ones genes, whereas the other 80 percent is dictated by one's lifestyle. In 2004, Dan Buettner, CEO of Blue Zones LLC, was determined to uncover the specific aspects of lifestyle and environment that led to longevity. By teaming up with National Geographic and the National Institute on Aging, Dan and his team found the five demographically confirmed, geographically defined areas with the highest percentage of centenarians (Loma Linda, California, US; Nicoya, Costa Rica; Sardinia, Italy; Ikaria, Greece; and Okinawa, Japan). These five areas were located using epidemiological data, statistics, birth certificates, and other research. Once these areas were established, they sent in a team of anthropologists, demographers, epidemiologists, and researchers to identify the lifestyle characteristics that might explain longevity. Many individuals have the capacity to make it well into the early nineties and largely without chronic disease. Blue Zones uncovered nine evidence-based common denominators among the world's centenarians that are believed to slow this aging process.

1. MOVE NATURALLY

The world's longest-lived people do not pump iron, run marathons, or join gyms. Instead, they live in environments that constantly nudge them into moving without thinking about it. They grow gardens and do not have mechanical conveniences for house and yard work.

2. PURPOSE

The Okinawans call it Ikigai, and the Nicoyans call it plan de vida. For both, it translates to "why I wake up in the morning." Knowing your sense of purpose is worth up to seven years of extra life expectancy.

3. DOWNSHIFT

Even people in the Blue Zones experience stress. Stress

leads to chronic inflammation, associated with every major age-related disease. The world's longest-lived people have routines to shed that stress. Okinawans take a few moments each day to remember their ancestors; Adventists pray; Ikarians take a nap; and Sardinians do happy hour.

4. 80 PERCENT RULE

"Hara hachi bu" – the Okinawan 2,500-year-old Confucian mantra said before meals reminds them to stop eating when their stomachs are 80 percent full. The 20 percent gap between not being hungry and feeling full could be the difference between losing weight or gaining it. People in the Blue Zones eat their smallest meal in the late afternoon or early evening and then they do not eat any more the rest of the day.

5. PLANT SLANT

Beans, including fava, black, soy, and lentils, are the cornerstone of most centenarian diets. Meat – mostly pork – is eaten on average only five times per month. Serving sizes are three to four ounces.

6. WINE

Most people in all Blue Zones drink one to two glasses per day with friends and/ or with food at 5:00 p.m. Moderate drinkers outlive nondrinkers.

7. BELONG

All but five of the 263 centenarians interviewed belonged to some faith-based community. Research shows that attending faith-based services four times per month will add four to fourteen years of life expectancy.

8. LOVED ONES FIRST

Successful centenarians in the Blue Zones put their families first. This means keeping aging parents and grandparents nearby or in the home. (It lowers disease and mortality rates of children in the home too.) They commit to a life partner (which can add up to three years of life expectancy) and invest in their children with time and love.

9. RIGHT TRIBE

The world's longest-lived people chose – or were born into – social circles that supported healthy behaviors, Okinawans created moais – groups of five friends that committed to each other for life. Research from the Framingham Studies shows that smoking, obesity, happiness, and even loneliness are contagious. The social networks of long-lived people favorably shaped their health behaviors.

In summary, it is important to select where and what kind of lifestyle we want to live. It is abundantly clear that we need to be involved and committed to work toward the creation of governmental policies for more sustainable environments for the aging and develop and maintain partnerships with governments, large employers, and other entities to improve lives and communities nationwide.

5

THE ENVIRONMENT AND ITS EFFECTS ON AGING

"The single biggest threat to our planet is the destruction of habitat and along the way loss of precious wildlife. We need to reach a balance where people, habitat, and wildlife can co-exist — if we don't everyone loses... one day."
— Steve Irwin

According to the World Health Organization, "Air pollution is now the world's largest single environmental health risk." Air pollution threatens the health of people in many parts of the world. New estimates in 2018 reveal that nine out of ten people breathe air containing high levels of pollutants. Both ambient (outdoor) and household (indoor) air pollution are responsible for about 7 million deaths globally per year; in the Western Pacific Region alone, around 2.2 million people die each year. There are other types of pollution too, such as waste. Our planet is currently facing climate change, deforestation, pollution, loss of biodiversity, oceanic dead zones, and overpopulation.

In this chapter, you will learn about air pollution and Alzheimer's risks as well as how clean air matters for a healthy brain. Certain environmental factors, like exposure to toxic chemicals and brain injury, have long been known to increase the risk of Alzheimer's, dementia, and Parkinson's.

James, one of my clients in China, told me that the air

pollution is the third leading mortality risk factor in China, with 1.1 million attributable deaths, 56 percent of which are caused by cardiovascular diseases. James, who travels for business between New York City and Beijing, suffers from eye and throat irritation and colds. Air pollution in China is causing significantly negative health effects. The issue is fueled by China's transition to an aging society with a climbing population of elders characterized by great physiological and social vulnerability.

Also, the rapid growth in the number of older Americans has many implications for public health, including the need to better understand the risks posed to older adults by environmental exposures. Biologic capacity declines with normal aging; this may be exacerbated in individuals with pre-existing health conditions. The environmental factors that accelerate aging are those that influence either damage of cellular macromolecules or interfere with their repair. Prominent among these are chronic inflammation, chronic infection, some metallic chemicals, ultraviolet light, and others that heighten oxidative stress.

Alzheimer's disease is one of those conditions where genetics is known to play a profound role but is not the sole factor in disease development and progression. The evidence is mounting that the environment has a great deal to do with the development of this neurodegenerative disorder. Moreover, it is now known that the right kind of nutrition and lifestyle may play preventive role in many cases. Dementia is a term used to describe a group of symptoms affecting memory, thinking, and social abilities severely enough to interfere with your daily life. Parkinson's disease is a progressive nervous system disorder that affects movement. Symptoms start gradually, sometimes starting with a barely noticeable tremor in just one hand. Tremors are common, but the disorder also commonly causes stiffness or slowing of movement.

A history of neurodegenerative diseases does not necessarily mean that a person will develop mental decline.

Neurodegenerative diseases are still highly preventable. By avoiding triggers in the environment and living a healthy, active life, one may expect to remain mentally alert until ripe old age. Neurodegenerative disease is caused by the progressive loss of structure or function of neurons, in the process known as neurodegeneration. Such neuronal damage may ultimately involve cell death. There's no single "miracle cure" for memory problems or other brain changes that come with aging. But there is cause for optimism. Science points to a combination of social factors and healthy habits that – taken together – can help you build, preserve, and protect your brain's function over time.

Experts used to think brain development peaked in late adolescence and it was all downhill from there. They believed if a person lost brain cells due to problems like a head injury, stroke, or substance abuse, nothing could be done to restore memory and brain function. Now, thanks to discoveries in neuroscience, we know that the brain can grow new cells and form new neural connections. Like our muscles and other body parts, the brain can rebuild itself through repeated use and exercise. This is great news for people who intend to live a long time. It means we can prevent memory loss by focusing on mental, physical, and social activities that promote healthy brain development such as getting enough sleep, exercise, meditation, hydration, cutting on stress and learning something new.

Even people with Alzheimer's disease and other dementias can benefit from a healthy lifestyle. It may help to think about your brain as a reservoir, gathering rainfall for use over time. The process starts before birth as the brain begins to develop, collecting "reserves" to spend later. The exchange continues throughout life, as your brain responds to your experiences and environment.

James Giordano, PhD, a professor of neurology and biochemistry at Georgetown University, told Healthline that a healthy brain can remain fully capable for the majority of a person's life span. "As a matter of fact, as we age, the neural nodes and networks formed throughout our life can become more efficient in their ability to link and relate prior and current experience to predictive decisions."

Giordano said there are two important adages that apply to the brain's network capabilities: effectiveness and efficiency. "First is that 'nerve cells that fire together, wire together,' which means that neurological nodes and networks are formed as a consequence of engagement and use," Giordano told Healthline. "Second, is that 'if you don't use it, you tend to lose it.' With life experience that comes with aging, we form and fortify certain neurological networks, and while we retain many – such as those involved in the performance of fundamental abilities, tasks, and skills, and basic concepts that are part of the repertoires of our life – other network connectivity weaken with disuse."

But just because we go through periods of inaction doesn't mean the brain can't rally. "The good news is that a healthy brain retains much of its capacity to reestablish and form node and network connectivity throughout much of the life span, well into old age," Giordano said. "It just requires the necessary stimuli to keep these mechanisms and processes actively engaged… This is why lifelong 'brain health' is so important."

Dr. Eric Larson, executive director at Kaiser Permanente, Washington Health Research Institute, recommends the following to keep your brain healthy.

1. Exercise regularly.
   Daily physical exercise has been shown to prevent or postpone your risk for Alzheimer's disease and other dementias. As little as fifteen to thirty minutes a day can make a difference.
2. If you smoke, quit.
   Tobacco use can harm all your organs, including your brain. But stopping now improves your chances for healthier brain function in the future, even if you've smoked for many years.
3. Take care of your heart and brain.

A healthy brain requires a good cardiovascular system. If you have high blood pressure, high cholesterol, diabetes, or atrial fibrillation, follow your doctor's advice.

4. Avoid a high-sugar diet.
High blood sugar can increase your risk for dementia, even without diabetes. Avoid highly sweetened foods like sodas and candy.

5. Keep your mind stimulated.
Games and puzzles are great. But also consider volunteer and social activities that keep you independent and engaged with friends and family. For example, learn new computer skills; participate on a board, in a book club, or dance group; or try gardening, crafts, or cooking.

6. Avoid certain drugs.
Talk to your doctor about your medication – both prescription and nonprescription. For brain health, you want to avoid dangerous interactions or being over-medicated.

7. Moderate or avoid alcohol.
Drinking has a stronger effect on our bodies as we age. Experts advise a limit of one drink per day for women and two drinks per day for men.

8. Prevent falls.
Falls can cause a head injury, broken bones, or other harm that triggers gradual or sudden loss of function. To avoid falling, practice balance and strength exercises. Beware that drinking and drugs can affect balance. And watch for uneven walking surfaces and cords that can trip you. Wear shoes or slippers with good soles. Avoid going barefoot or walking in stocking feet. If you bike or ski, wear a helmet.

9. Minimize stress.
Hormones secreted when you're under stress have a stronger effect on older brains, challenging your

ability to recover from emotional upset. Take change slowly and learn ways to cope with anxiety or tension.

10. Sleep well.

Inadequate sleep is linked to slower thinking and the risk of dementia. Seven to nine hours a night is best. But be wary of sleep medications that can make cognitive problems worse. Instead, talk to your doctor about habits to help your body settle down at bedtime.

Dr. Bradley Katz, a professor and neuro-ophthalmologist at the University of Utah, said, "Keeping our brains in tip-top shape as we age doesn't only mean learning new things or doing brain puzzles to keep the brain stimulated. It also means maintaining a healthy diet to support our brain health and our overall physical health, exercising regularly, quitting smoking, and controlling cholesterol levels to maintain good blood flow to the brain."

A healthy brain needs fifteen dietary components, including ten "brain-healthy" food groups: green leafy vegetables, other vegetables, nuts, berries, beans, whole grains, fish, poultry, olive oil, and resveratrol, a supplement derived from red wine.

Dr. Verna R. Porter, a neurologist and the director of programs for dementia, Alzheimer's disease, and neurocognitive disorders at the Pacific Brain Health Center, Providence Saint John's Medical Center, in Santa Monica, California, said that "chronic or persistent stress can lead to nerve cell decline and even death, which may manifest as atrophy (shrinkage in size) of important memory areas in the brain... Nerve cell dysfunction and degeneration in turn increases the risk of Alzheimer's disease and dementia. Studies have shown that regular meditation, prayer, reflection, and religious practice may diminish the damaging effects of stress on the brain."

Absolutely, we need to reach a balance where people, habitat, and wildlife can coexist. I am encouraged that the

United Nations' 17 Sustainable Development Goals (SDGs) are part of a plan to target the most extreme poverty and tyranny through development, all while taking our planet into greater consideration.

Goal Number One – No Poverty: End poverty in all its forms everywhere. More than 700 million people still live in extreme poverty on less than USD $1.90 a day. They struggle to fulfill the most basic needs (health, education, access to water and sanitation). Most of them – more than 400 million – live in sub-Saharan Africa. An estimated 71 million additional people around the world will be pushed into extreme poverty due to COVID-19, the first rise in global poverty since 1998. Poverty affects developed countries as well. Right now, 30 million children are growing up poor in the world's richest countries. Eradicating poverty in all its forms remains one of the greatest challenges facing humanity. While the number of people living in extreme poverty dropped by more than half between 1990 and 2015 – from 1.9 billion to 731 million – too many are still struggling for the most basic human needs.

Goal Number Two – Zero Hunger: End hunger, achieve food security, and improved nutrition and promote sustainable agriculture. More than 750 million people suffer from hunger worldwide, the vast majority in developing countries. This number is expected to go up by over 100 million in 2020 alone due to COVID-19. Hunger and malnutrition are barriers to sustainable development because hungry people are less productive, more prone to disease, and less able to improve their livelihoods. To nourish today's 750 million hungry people and the additional 2 billion people expected by 2050, a profound change of the global food and agriculture system is needed. To end all forms of hunger and malnutrition by 2030 and ensure that all people – especially children – have access to sufficient and nutritious food all year round requires promoting sustainable agricultural practices, such as supporting small scale farmers and allowing equal access to land, technology, and markets.

International cooperation is also necessary to provide investment in infrastructure and technology that improves agricultural productivity.

Goal Number Three – Good Health and Well-Being: Ensure healthy lives and promote wellbeing for all at all ages. Despite great strides in improving people's health in recent years, inequalities in health care access still persist. The COVID-19 pandemic is throwing progress even further off track. More than five million children die before their fifth birthday every year. 16,000 children die each day from preventable diseases such as measles and tuberculosis. Every day, hundreds of women die during pregnancy or from childbirth related complications. These deaths can be avoided through prevention and treatment, education, immunization campaigns, and sexual and reproductive healthcare. The Sustainable Development Goals (SDGs) make a bold commitment to end the epidemics of AIDS, tuberculosis, malaria, and other communicable diseases by 2030. The aim is to achieve universal health coverage and provide access to safe and affordable medicines and vaccines for all.

Goal Number Four – Quality Education: Ensure inclusive and equitable quality education and promote lifelong learning opportunities for all. Enormous progress has been made in achieving the target of universal primary education with 91 percent enrollment in 2015. However, 258 million children and youth of age 6 to 17 were still out of school in 2018, and more than half of children and adolescents are not meeting minimum proficiency standards in reading and mathematics. In 2020, as schools closed due to COVID-19, an estimated 90 percent of all students were out of school, with at least 500 million of those left without access to distance learning options. In addition to free primary and secondary schooling for all boys and girls by 2030, the aim is to provide equal access to affordable vocational training, eliminate gender and wealth disparities, and achieve universal access to quality higher education. Education is the key that will allow many other Sustainable Development Goals to be achieved. When people can get quality education, they can break from the cycle of poverty. Education helps to reduce inequalities and to reach gender equality. It also empowers people everywhere to live more healthy and sustainable lives. Education is also crucial to fostering tolerance between people and contributes to more peaceful societies.

Goal Number Five – Gender Equality: Achieve gender equality and empower all women and girls. Women and girls represent half of the world's population and, therefore, also half of its potential. But gender inequality persists everywhere and stagnates social progress. On average, women in the labor market still earn 23 percent less than men globally. On average, women spend about three times as many hours in unpaid domestic and care work as men. Sexual violence and exploitation, the unequal division of unpaid care and domestic work, and discrimination in public office all remain huge barriers. All these areas of inequality have been exacerbated by the COVID-19 pandemic. There has been a surge in reports of sexual violence, women have taken on more care work due to school closures, and 70 percent of health and social workers globally are women. As of 2014, 143 countries have guaranteed equality between men and women in their constitutions, but 52 have yet to take this step. Gender equality is not only a fundamental human right, but a necessary foundation for a peaceful, prosperous, and sustainable world.

Goal Number Six – Clean Water and Sanitation: Ensure availability and sustainable management of water and sanitation for all. Access to water, sanitation and hygiene is a human right. Yet billions are still faced with daily challenges accessing even the most basic of services. Water scarcity affects more than 40 percent of the world population and is projected to increase with the rise of global temperatures as a result of climate change. Globally, three in ten people lack access to safely managed drinking water services. And six in ten people lack access to safely managed sanitation facilities, leaving an estimated three billion people without basic handwashing facilities at home, a critical need to prevent infection and contain the spread of COVID-19. Investments in infrastructure and sanitation facilities, protection and restoration of water-related ecosystems, and hygiene education are among the steps necessary to ensure universal access to safe and affordable drinking water for all by 2030.

Goal Number Seven – Affordable and Clean Energy: Our everyday life depends on reliable and affordable energy. And yet the consumption of energy is the dominant contributor to climate change, accounting for around 60 percent of total global greenhouse gas emissions. From 2000 to 2018, the proportion of the global population with access to electricity has increased from 78 percent to 90 percent. In the least developed countries, that proportion has more than doubled during the same period. And yet there are still about 789 million people around the with no access to electricity. Ensuring universal access to affordable electricity by 2030 means investing in clean energy sources such as solar, wind and thermal. Expanding infrastructure and upgrading technology to provide clean energy in all developing countries is a crucial goal that can both encourage growth and help the environment.

Goal Number Eight– Decent Work and Economic Growth: Promote sustained, inclusive, and sustainable economic growth, full and productive employment, and decent work for all. Globally, labor productivity has increased, and the unemployment rate has decreased. However, more progress is needed to increase employment opportunities, especially for young people, reduce informal employment and labour market inequality (particularly in terms of the gender pay gap), promote safe and secure working environments, and improve access to financial services to ensure sustained and inclusive economic growth. The global unemployment rate in 2019 was 5 percent, down from 6.4 percent in 2000. However, COVID-19 could cause the equivalent of 400 million job losses in 2020, depending on the policy measures adopted. The pandemic will have a particularly adverse impact on workers in the informal economy, where an estimated 1.6 billion workers risk being impacted. A persistent lack of decent work opportunities, insufficient investments and under-consumption contribute to the erosion of the basic social contract: that all must share in progress. The creation of quality jobs remains a major challenge for almost all economies.

Goal Number Nine – Industry, Innovation, and Infrastructure: Build resilient infrastructure, promote inclusive and sustainable industrialization and foster innovation. Some progress has been made in the manufacturing industry. The global share of manufacturing value added in Gross Domestic Product (GDP) increased from 15.2 percent in 2005 to 16.5 percent in 2018. However, the share of manufacturing in least developed countries remains low, posing a serious challenge to the target of doubling industry's share of GDP by 2030. Global manufacturing slowed in both developing and developed regions in 2018–2019, mainly attributed to emerging trade and tariff barriers that constrain investment and future growth and has plummeted in 2020 because of the pandemic. While global internet coverage has expanded widely, as of 2019, 46 percent of the global population still does not use the internet. Investments in infrastructure – transport, irrigation, energy and information and communication technology – are crucial to achieving sustainable development and empowering communities in many countries.

Goal Number Ten – Reduce inequality within and among countries: Income inequality is on the rise – particularly within countries. As of 2017, the richest 10 percent earn at least 20 percent of total global income. The poorest 40 percent earn less than 25 percent of total global income. On average, and considering population size, inequality has increased by 11 percent in developing countries between 1990 and 2010. Inequality threatens long-term social and economic development, harms poverty reduction, and destroys people's sense of fulfillment and self-worth. To reduce inequality, policies should be universal and pay special attention to the needs of disadvantaged and marginalized populations, which will be disproportionately affected by the economic impacts of COVID-19.

Goal Number Eleven – Sustainable Cities and Communities: Make cities and human settlements inclusive, safe, resilient, and sustainable. Half of the world's population live in cities. By 2050, 6.5 billion people – two-thirds of humanity – will live in urban areas. In the developing world, the rapid growth of cities, along wit the increasing rural to urban migration, has led to a boom in mega-cities. In 1990, there were ten mega-cities with 10 million inhabitants or more. In 2014, there are 28 mega-cities, home to a total of 453 million people. This rapid urbanization outpaces the development of housing, infrastructure, and services, which led to a rise in the share of the urban population living in slums – 24 percent in 2018. As the COVID-19 pandemic has made clear, sustainable development cannot be achieved without significantly transforming the way urban spaces are built and managed. Making cities safe and sustainable means ensuring access to safe and affordable housing, upgrading slum settlements, investing in public transport, creating green spaces, and improving urban planning and management in a way that is both participatory and inclusive.

Goal Number Twelve– Responsible Consumption and Production: Ensure sustainable consumption and production patterns. If the global population reaches 9.8 billion by 2050, the equivalent of almost three planets will be required to provide the natural resources needed to sustain current lifestyles. In 2015, almost twelve tons of resources were extracted per person, with electronic waste as the fastest-growing sector. This means that production, consumption, and natural resources must be managed better and differently. The world's ecological footprint should be reduced by changing the way goods and resources are produced and consumed. Shared natural resources should be managed efficiently, and toxic waste and pollutants disposed of carefully. Support should be provided to developing countries to move towards more sustainable patterns of consumption by 2030.

Goal Number Thirteen – Climate Action: Take urgent action to combat climate change and its impacts. Climate change affects every country on every continent. It is caused by human activities and threatens the future of our planet. With rising greenhouse gas emissions, climate change is occurring at rates much faster than anticipated and its effects are clearly felt worldwide. The impacts include changing weather patterns, rising sea level, and more extreme weather events. The year 2019 was the second warmest on record, bringing with it massive wildfires, hurricanes, droughts, floods, and other climate disasters. If left unchecked, climate change will undo a lot of the progress made over the past years in development. It will also provoke mass migrations that will lead to instability and wars. Affordable, scalable solutions are now available to enable countries to leapfrog to cleaner, more resilient, and lower-carbon economies. Climate change is a global challenge that requires coordinated international cooperation.

Goal Number Fourteen – Life Below Water: Conserve and sustainably use the oceans, seas, and marine resources for sustainable development. Oceans cover three quarters of the Earth's surface, contain 97 percent of the Earth's water, and represent 99 percent of the living space on the planet by volume. The world's oceans provide key natural resources, including food, medicines, biofuels, and other products; help with the breakdown and removal of waste and pollution; and to use coastal ecosystems as buffers to reduce damage from storms. Today, more than 30 percent of the world's fish stocks are overexploited, and marine pollution is reaching alarming levels, with an average of 13,000 pieces of plastic litter to be found on every square kilometer of ocean. Careful management of this essential global resource is a key feature of a sustainable future.

Goal Number Fifteen – Life on Land: Protect, restore, and promote sustainable use of terrestrial ecosystems; sustainably manage forests; combat desertification; halt and reverse land degradation; and halt biodiversity loss. Plant life provides 80 percent of the human diet, and agriculture is an important economic resource and means of development. Forests cover more than 30 percent of the Earth's surface, but seven million hectares of forests are being lost every year, while the persistent degradation of drylands has led to the desertification of close to four billion hectares. Of the 8,300 animal breeds known, 8 percent are extinct, and 22 percent are at risk of extinction. Wildlife trafficking also disrupts ecosystems and contributes to the spread of infectious diseases, such as COVID-19. Halting deforestation and restoring the use of terrestrial ecosystems is necessary to reduce the loss of natural habitats and biodiversity which are part of our common heritage.

Goal Number Sixteen – Peace, Justice, and Strong Institutions: Promote peaceful and inclusive societies for sustainable development, provide access to justice for all, and build effective, accountable, and inclusive institutions at all levels. People everywhere should be free of fear from all forms of violence and feel safe as they go about their lives whatever their ethnicity, faith, or sexual orientation. High levels of armed violence and insecurity have a destructive impact on a country's development. Sexual violence, crime, exploitation, and torture are prevalent where there is conflict or no rule of law, and countries must take measures to protect those who are most at risk. Governments, civil society, and communities need to work together to find lasting solutions to conflict and insecurity. Strengthening the rule of law and promoting human rights is key to this process, as is reducing the flow of illicit arms, combating corruption, and always ensuring inclusive participation.

Goal Number Seventeen – Partnerships for the Goals: Strengthen the means of implementation and revitalize the global partnership for sustainable development. The 2030 Agenda for Sustainable Development is universal and calls for action by all countries – developed and developing – to ensure no one is left behind. It requires partnerships between governments, the private sector, and civil society. The Sustainable Development Goals can only be realized with a strong commitment to global partnership and cooperation. Significant challenges remain: official development assistance is declining; private investment flows are not well aligned with sustainable development, there continues to be a significant digital divide, and there are ongoing trade tensions. To be successful, everyone will need to mobilize both existing and additional resources and developed countries will need to fulfill their official development assistance commitments.

These SDGs, established by the United Nations, are an urgent call for action by all countries in global partnership and represent benchmarks for a better world and environment for everyone. All these seventeen sustainable goals are important for humanity's overall wellbeing. And since this chapter is about the environment and its effects on aging, I would like to share with you and invite you to actively participate in the successful accomplishment of Sustainable Goals 13, 14, and 15. If you are interested in making a difference, click on the link below for volunteer opportunities. Thank you.

https://www.un.org/en/academic-impact/work4un-un-volunteers

Recently, the United Nations scientists delivered a stark warning about the impact of climate change on people and the planet, saying that ecosystem collapse, species extinction, deadly heatwaves, and floods are among the "unavoidable multiple climate hazards" the world will face over the next two decades due to global warming. "This report is a dire warning about the consequences of inaction," said Hoesung Lee, chair of the Intergovernmental Panel on Climate Change (IPCC). According to the report, human-induced climate change is causing dangerous and widespread disruption in nature and affecting billions of lives all over the world, despite efforts to reduce the risks, with people and ecosystems least able to cope being hardest hit.

In summary, the environment and its effect on aging is real! If you are not yet involved in your community and/ or if you want to make a difference and help save humankind and Planet Earth, visit https://actnow.aworld.org/.

6

LIFESTYLE INCLUDING LAUGHTER, MUSIC, FUN, AND SEX

"Music gives a soul to the universe, wings to the mind, flight
to the imagination, and life to everything."
— Plato

In this chapter, you will learn how therapeutic music and laughing have been clinically proven to improve sleep, relieve stress, calm and soothe your pet, and give you more energy for your day, impacting longevity. Therapeutic music is intended to alleviate a physical, emotional, or mental concern. Common usage of the term usually refers to acoustic music played or sung live in a variety of healthcare settings, to enhance the healing atmosphere. There is a great deal of research about how music can be therapeutic to older adults. According to the American Music Therapy Association, music can provide memory recall which contributes to reminiscence and satisfaction with life.

Music and laughter can bring lasting benefits to your state of mind. Music provides positive changes in mood and emotional state. As I am writing this chapter, I am reminded of Tony Bennett and Lady Gaga's successful live concert honoring their musical legacy and their enduring friendship. They performed two sold-out shows at Radio City Music Hall in August 2021 to celebrate Bennett's ninety-fifth birthday. What is amazing is how, at ninety-five years old, Tony, who has Alzheimer's disease, was able to remember every single word of all the music they performed at this amazing live concert performance.

Tony's Alzheimer's disease is the most common form of age-related dementia. Alzheimer's is characterized by a progressive memory loss that robs its sufferers of many of the gifts that we all take for granted – speech, understanding, treasured memories, recognition of loved ones – and leaves them utterly dependent on caregivers. This is a great example of how music gives wings to the mind, flight to the imagination, and life to everything.

Laughter is a potent releaser of endorphins. Recent research has shown that when you take the time to relax, laugh, play, and have fun, you become healthier, happier, more creative, and more resilient to life's setbacks. When you choose to have fun, to let go and laugh, your physiology changes. Your blood pressure drops, your glands release natural pain-killing hormones, and your tensely held muscles finally let go and relax. You even become more effective and productive at work if you find time for lighthearted fun during your busy days and weeks. I cannot imagine what our relationships would be like without laughter. One of my life goals is to laugh and play a little each day. If you have not laughed at yourself or some situation during the day, then watch a funny sitcom or read something funny before you retire to bed at night. You need something to lighten the day and to remind you that life is as fun as you choose to make it.

It turns out there is some scientific veracity behind the adage, Laughter is the best medicine. Laughter activates the body's natural relaxation response. "It's like internal jogging, providing a good massage to all internal organs while also toning abdominal muscles," according to Dr. Gulshan Sethi, head of cardiothoracic surgery at the Tucson Medical Center and faculty at the University of Arizona's Center for Integrative Medicine. Perhaps that's why Deepak Chopra says the healthiest response to life is laughter. Studies have found that laughter can have healing properties, and it's contagious.

When you're feeling down, finding friends to laugh with can help your brain trigger its own laughter response and foster closeness, both of which contribute to your sense of wellbeing. Why do you think that sense of humor is such an important trait when looking for a partner? We like the feeling of shared laughter, and our body wants as much of this feeling as possible. When you laugh, there's a contraction of muscles, which increases blood flow and oxygenation. This stimulates the heart and lungs and triggers the release of endorphins that help you to feel more relaxed both physically and emotionally.

According to one study done at Indiana State School of nursing, mirthful laughter may increase the level of natural killer cells, a type of white blood cell that attacks cancer cells. People who are resilient are happier and more successful. The ability to acknowledge mistakes without becoming angry or frustrated plays an important role in developing resilience. Laughing at mistakes allows us to recognize that making errors is a part of being human. Make humor a priority by reading a funny book, watching a comedy, or listening to your favorite comedian. Share laughter with friends. Spend more time with people who have fun. The ability to laugh at yourself makes you attractive to others and can help relieve your stress. Focus on finding the laughable moments in your day and then tell a friend your funny story to increase the power of laughter by sharing. Be discerning about your humor by laughing with – not at – people. Your ability to laugh can be cultivated with practice so start by prioritizing fun. Find occasions to be silly, and remember that laughter like smiling is never depleted when you share it.

The recent results obtained by researchers from the University of Oxford in England and Aalto University in Finland have revealed how social laughter leads to endorphin release in the brain, possibly promoting the establishment of social bonds. Social laughter led to pleasurable feelings and significantly increased release of endorphins and other opioid peptides in the brain areas controlling arousal and emotions. The more opioid receptors the participants had in their brains, the more they laughed during the experiment. The researchers highlighted that endorphin release induced by social laughter may be an important pathway that supports the formation, reinforcement, and maintenance of social bonds between humans. The pleasurable and calming effects of the endorphin release might signal safety and promote feelings of togetherness.

The relationship between opioid receptor density and laughter rate also suggests that the opioid system may underlie individual differences in sociability, said Professor Lauri Nummenmaa from the University of Turku in Finland. The results emphasize the importance of vocal communication in maintaining human social networks. Other primates maintain social contacts by mutual grooming, which also induces endorphin release. This is, however, very time consuming. Because social laughter leads to similar chemical response in the brain, this allows significant expansion of human social networks: laughter is highly contagious, and the endorphin response may thus easily spread through large groups that laugh together, tells Professor Robin Dunbar from the University of Oxford. Laughing with friends releases endorphins (the chemicals that help us to feel good) in our brains via opioid receptors. Therapeutic music has been clinically proven to improve sleep, relieve stress, calm, soothe your pet, and gain more energy for your day.

In a 2007 New England Journal of Medicine study of a representative sample of the U.S. population, Dr. Stacy Tessler Lindau, a professor of obstetrics-gynecology and geriatrics at the University of Chicago, and colleagues surveyed more than 3,000 older adults, single and partnered, about sex (defined as "any mutually voluntary activity with another person that involves sexual contact, whether or not intercourse or orgasm occurs"). They found that 53 percent of participants ages sixty-five to seventy-four had sex at least once in the previous year. In the seventy-five to eighty-five age group, only 26 percent did. (Lindau notes that a major determinant of sexual activity is whether one has a partner or not – and many older people are widowed, separated, or divorced.)

Older people may want and need to be close to others as they grow older. For some, this includes the desire to continue an active, satisfying sex life. With aging, that may mean adapting the sexual activity to accommodate physical, health, and other changes. There are many ways to have sex and be intimate alone or with a partner. The expression of your sexuality could include many types of touch or stimulation. Some adults may choose not to engage in sexual activity, and that's also normal. According to the National Institute of Aging, here are some of the common problems older adults may face with sex. Normal aging brings physical changes in both men and women. These changes sometimes affect the ability to have and enjoy sex.

Talk with your partner about these changes and how you are feeling. Your doctor may have suggestions to help have sex easier. Also, some illnesses, disabilities, medicines, and surgeries can affect your ability to have and enjoy sex. There are things you can do on your own for an active and enjoyable sex life. If you have a long-term partner, take time to enjoy each other and to understand the changes you both are facing. Talk to your partner or partners about your needs. You may find that affection – hugging, kissing, touching, and spending time together – can be just what you need or a path to greater intimacy and sex.

There are advantages and disadvantages of growing older. I have shared with you some of the disadvantages on the preceding paragraphs. Some of the advantages of growing older may include having an epiphany that some of the things you once thought were critical – and perhaps even matters of life or death – really don't matter much at all. You now have enough hard-won experience to know that things have a way of working themselves out in their time. Rather than fear missing what other people are doing, you are entirely happy to just do whatever makes you feel comfortable and relaxed – without the need to follow the crowd. Who says you're ever too old to try new things? In fact, this can be an ideal time to make a fun shift. This is the perfect time to take your decades of accomplishments, all your skill sets and passions, and co-mingle them in new and interesting ways. I am enjoying seeing my extended family grow, having fun with my granddaughter Maven Rose, learning, reading interesting books, mentoring, and doing enjoyable non-profit work that is in alignment with my values to promote pay equity and equity for women and girls. As we age and gain more wisdom, we can appreciate what matters to us that may not have occurred to us in the frenetic days of youth. The quality of our personal and business relationships and our precious time left to enjoy them.

In summary, surround yourself with people that you love and the things that bring you happiness. Live life on your own terms and appreciate the fleeting nature of time and the power of love.

7

EAT LESS, LIVE LONGER

*"The secret of living well and longer is eat half, walk double,
laugh triple and love without measure."*
— Tibetan Proverb

In this chapter, I will teach you some ideas about how to increase your wellness with food that you enjoy. It is important to eat a variety of colorful foods to receive a broad spectrum of nutrients. The six basic nutrients in meals are proteins, water, fats, carbohydrates, minerals, and vitamins. Proteins, carbohydrates, and fats provide energy. Proteins form important parts of the body's main structural components and have a major role in building and repairing. Carbohydrates are the body's preferred source of energy. Fats (lipids), in addition to providing the most concentrated form of energy, play a role in the storage and transportation of fat-soluble vitamins. Minerals and vitamins regulate body functions.

Deep pigments in plant foods are dense with nutrients and generally have more antioxidants. Cook with color to add visual appeal and encourage appreciation of a meal. Enhance your health with phytochemicals (plant chemicals) that have protective or disease-preventive properties. Some of the benefits include protection against oxidative damage and decreased risk of cancer and heart disease. The easiest way to get more phytochemicals is to eat more fruit and vegetables.

Robert, one of my clients who frequently suffered from indigestion and a bad skin condition, at my suggestion, implemented the Ayurvedic lifestyle and started eating his biggest meal in the middle of the day when his agni (digestive power) is the strongest. Instead of eating his largest meal late at night after coming home tired from work and falling sleep immediately while watching his favorite TV program, Robert changed his eating habits and started enjoying his biggest meal at noon followed by a short walk to help with his digestion. Robert also started to drink more water and avoided overeating and reducing ice-cold foods and sweet beverages. This small eating and behavioral change helped to minimize my client's indigestion and skin condition.

What is agni? It is the metabolic power responsible for extracting nourishment and eliminating toxins. Your health depends on proper digestion. When our digestive fire is strong and healthy, we can easily digest food and experiences. We extract the greatest level of nourishment from our diet (ojas). Yogapedia's definition of ojas is "vigor." In the practice of Ayurveda, ojas is thought to be responsible for vitality, strength, health, length of life, immunity, and mental/ emotional wellness. When our digestive fire is weak or irregular, we cannot properly digest even potentially nourishing substances, and our body starts to accumulate toxins (ama). We keep agni strong by eating the proper amount; eating the right foods; and managing stress, which can dampen agni.

What is microbiome? The microbiome is a vast colony of micro-organisms that inhabit our body, including bacteria and other microbes. These microbes live mainly in our digestive tracts, in our mouths, and even on our skin. The microbiome is beneficial for our health; it helps to digest our food, regulate hormones and immune system, and influence our nervous system and emotions. In your daily life, the choices you make about what you eat can make the greatest difference in cultivating a healthy gut microbiome. You need to avoid refined and processed foods and favor fresh, real food. You can be assured that you are nurturing your microbiome, body, and mind with the highest-quality, anti-inflammatory nutritive.

There are five primary elements of life or building blocks of nature that make up everything we perceive through our senses – Space, Air, Fire, Water and Earth – which exist both within us and in the world around us. In Ayurvedic medicine, there are three energies (doshas) believed to circulate in the body and govern physiological activity. The three doshas are derived from the five elements. The five elements organize themselves into three essential principles of life: movement, metabolism, and structure, known in Sanskrit as Vata, Pitta, and Kapha. These principles, which we can think of as air, fire, and earth, are the forces that govern every natural function and regulate every process within our mind and body. Since each of us is a unique expression of nature, we each have an inherent tendency toward one or more of these principles. This explains why we each responds so differently to the same stimulus. Some of us are naturally earthier, while others are more fiery or airy.

As we discuss the functions and characteristics of each of these principles, notice which ones you most identify with. Each of the mind-body principles – vata, pitta, and kapha – have a balanced expression and an out-of-balance expression. When these principles are circulating in the mind-body physiology in appropriate proportions, we feel healthy and happy, and all our bodily functions work in harmony with one another. Unhealthy lifestyle choices can imbalance the doshas. However, when we follow an improper diet and make unhealthy lifestyle choices, these principles may become disturbed and cause distress in mind or body. It is important to prepare nutritional foods to increase your wellness with food that you enjoy. It is important to remember to eat a variety of colorful foods to receive a broad spectrum of basic nutrients, including proteins, water, fats, carbohydrates, minerals, and vitamins

The Harvard Medical School recommends making the

following changes when it comes to creating a healthy diet that you can enjoy. Be relaxed about your diet. You will never find a perfect food. Not everything on your plate needs to have a higher purpose. Take your tastes and preferences into account. If beef is your favorite food, it is okay to eat it, but make it a Sunday treat instead of a daily staple.

Learn to think about food in a new way. Years ago, meat and potatoes were American ideals. Now we know that vegetables, fruits, whole grains, nuts, and fish are best for you. Experiment with new recipes and meal plans. Be creative and take chances. Instead of dreading your new diet, have fun with it.

Change slowly. Give yourself time to change, targeting one item a week. Start with breakfast, switching from eggs, bacon, donuts, white toast, or bagels to oatmeal or bran cereal and fruit. If you just can't spare ten minutes for a sit-down breakfast, grab high-fiber cereal bars instead of donuts or muffins. Try out salads, low-fat yogurt or low-fat cottage cheese, tuna or peanut butter sandwiches, and fruit for lunch. Snack on unsalted nuts, trail mix, fruit, raw veggies, Rye Krisp, or graham crackers. Try eating a few handfuls of a crunchy fiber cereal, such as Kashi, or nibble on a cereal bar. For dinner, experiment with fish, skinless poultry, beans, brown rice, whole-wheat pasta, and – of course – salads and veggies. Choose meats and poultry that are organic, grass fed, free range, hormone free, and antibiotic free. Fish should be wild, hormone free, and antibiotic free. Other healthy protein could include bison, herring, lamb, mackerel, shrimp, skinless chicken, skinless turkey, tuna and wild salmon. Fruit and low-fat frozen desserts are examples of desirable after-dinner treats. And there's nothing wrong with the occasional cake, pie, or chocolates if the portions are moderate.

If you are serious about making a change, consider ditching the following foods that are not good for your health and longevity.

- Bread, pasta, tortillas, and other foods that contain gluten
- Breakfast cereals (including oatmeal)
- Condiments, such as ketchup, soy sauce, and barbecuc sauce, that contain sugar, artificial ingredients, excessive salt, or gluten
- Corn (including popcorn, cornbread, and popped corn chips)
- Dairy foods such as milk, cheese, cream, yogurt, and ice cream
- Foods that contain genetically modified ingredients
- Foods that contain high-fructose corn syrup or trans (hydrogenated) fats
- Foods that contain sugar, artificial sweeteners, or soy
- Fruit juice (even 100 percent fresh)
- Grain-based foods (cereal, rice, instant oatmeal, wheat, barley, rye, and corn)
- Jams, jellies, pancake syrup
- Most cooking oils (corn, safflower, canola, soy)
- Processed frozen dinners
- Processed meats such as lunch meats
- Salty processed snacks (potato chips, popcorn, pretzels, nacho chips, crackers)
- Soy-based foods, such as protein bars, powders, oils and snack foods
- Sugary processed snacks (cakes, cookies, cupcakes, candy)
- Sweetened drinks, such as fruit punch, lemonade, and soda
- White potatoes
- Commercially raised beef and poultry
- Farm raised fish
- Pork and ham
- Processed lunch meats
- Processed meat such as bacon, sausage, pepperoni, and hot dogs

Diabetes, high blood pressure, heart attacks, strokes, and cancer are distressingly common. Many factors contribute to these complex problems, but the basic reasons are simple: we eat too much, we choose the wrong foods, and we don't get enough exercise. Scientists know what diet is best for health. The fine print has changed and is likely to change some more, but the key facts are in. Good eating is not a punishment but an opportunity. If you know why it's important and what to do, you'll find it enjoyable and satisfying. And if you establish an overall pattern of healthful nutrition, you'll have plenty of wiggle room to savor the treats that matter most to you.

Research indicates that moderate exercise, when practiced regularly, can roll back the clock on your DNA. Fill up your plate with vegetables. While there are numerous debates about the best diet for increased lifespan, nearly every diet agrees that eating more vegetables is the way to go. Also, consider intermittent fasting (with many variations on how this is achieved). Studies dating as far back as the 1930s have shown that caloric restriction extends the longevity of mice and other test species. It is important to get enough sleep. Most people feel best when they get seven to nine hours of sleep per night.

Carefully manage your stress. Stress can have unhealthy effects on your body and can promote unhealthy behaviors, such as overeating. Don't smoke or drink excessive amounts of alcohol. Make a commitment today to make one healthy change a week. Before you know, you'll be feeling better and on the road to longevity.

Cultivate personal relationships. Spending time with our loved ones does seem to improve longevity, maybe because it decreases stress or risky behaviors. One study led by researchers at the University of Exeter Medical School in England found that volunteers had a 22 percent reduction in mortality compared to non-volunteers.

If you are wondering what else contributes to a good life and how you can extend your life span, I will share with you the Harvard Study of Adult Development on what makes a good life and the lessons from the longest study on happiness. For seventy-five years, Harvard tracked the lives of 724 men, year after year, asking about their work, their home lives, their health, asking all along the way without knowing how their life stories were going to turn out. In a TEDx talk, psychiatrist Robert Waldinger shares important lessons learned from the study as well as some practical, old-as-the-hills wisdom on how to build a fulfilling, long life.

It turns out that people who are more socially connected to family, to friends, and to the community are happier. They're physically healthier, and they live longer than people who are less well connected. And the experience of loneliness turns out to be toxic. People who are more isolated than they want to be from others find that they are less happy, their health declines earlier in midlife, their brain functioning declines sooner, and they live shorter lives than people who are not lonely. And the sad fact is that at any given time, more than one in five Americans will report that they're lonely. Good relationships don't just protect our bodies; they protect our brains. It turns out that being in a securely attached relationship to another person is protective – the people who are in relationships where they feel they can count on the other person in times of need, those people's memories stay sharper longer. And the people in relationships where they feel they can't count on the other one, those are the people who experience earlier memory decline.

When it comes to love without measure, when it comes to mercy, it is always best to be on the merciful side. Shall you stop judging and condemning and enter a life of forgiveness? For the measure with which you measure will in return be measured out to you? We are challenged to love as we want to be loved.

"The measure of love is to love without measure."
— Francis De Sales

In our call to love, we must not be calculated. We must not hold back. Take a moment today and ask yourself what your motive to love is. Sometimes, we love for selfish reasons, to get something in return. Love without measure is calling us to simply love without wanting anything in return – to simply love for the sake of the other.

In closing, I leave you to reflect on this Marcus Aurelius quote: "Accept the things to which fate binds you, and love the people with whom fate brings you together but do so with all your heart."

8

INTERVENTIONS TO REDUCE AGING

"We are not victims of aging, sickness, and death. These are part of the scenery, not the seer, who is immune to any form of change. This seer is the spirit, the expression of eternal being."

— Deepak Chopra

Longevity must begin in early life, including taking care of your immune system, relieving stress and anxiety, and nourishing a healthy brain. Terrie Moffitt, university professor of psychology at Duke University, suggests that preventive interventions that aim to slow aging and extend healthspan must begin earlier in life. Because people who have early-onset mental disorders tend to be the same people who have multi-morbid physical diseases in later life, she says "improved mental health care might have a great opportunity to prevent the rising burden of age-related diseases."

Your immune system protects you; it detects germs that could make you sick and attacks them with antibodies. In autoimmune diseases, your immune system attacks a part of your body by mistake. In rheumatoid arthritis, the immune system attacks the joints. In inflammatory bowel disease, the immune system attacks the gastrointestinal tract. In autoimmune encephalitis (AE), the immune system attacks the brain. Alzheimer's disease, multiple sclerosis, autism, schizophrenia, and many other neurological and psychiatric conditions have been linked to inflammation in the brain.

There's growing evidence that immune cells and molecules play a key role in normal brain development and function as well.

Stress can be normal, especially since it is already part of our daily lives. When you experience stress, a part of your brain – specifically the hypothalamus – reacts, allowing the release of stress hormones. Stress hormones are the same hormones that make you sense the "fight or flight response" of your body. When you are threatened, stressed, or having an intense emotion, you will feel that your heart is beating fast, as your heart rate increases. Your breath also becomes faster, your muscles shake, and for some, it leads to uncontrollable shedding of tears.

Chronic stress can affect your body, both in terms of your physical health and mental health. If left untreated or unmanaged, it may result in consistent irritability, anxiety disorder, depression or major depressive disorder, insomnia, headache, back pain, shoulder pain, diarrhea, constipation, stomachache, and nausea and vomiting. For some, stress is diverted to overeating, substance abuse (including drugs, seaters, and alcohol), as well as social withdrawal. It can even lead to certain illnesses and serious health conditions like high blood pressure, stroke, heart attack, type 2 diabetes, heartburn or acid reflux, erectile dysfunction for males, and irregular, heavier, or more painful menstruation for females. Too much stress can result in chronic anxiety and depression. Yet it does not mean that we cannot control them anymore. Of course, stress can be normal or destructive.

As a Certified Chopra Health Instructor, I recommend the following ways to release stress:

1. Eating healthy, eating green goods, and avoiding processed junk foods. To relieve stress and anxiety be active during the day for a healthy sleep night.
2. Healthy sleeping is essential to functioning well during the day. Sleep restores your brain by repairing and reorganizing your memory and learning. The

best way to sleep is to make your room completely dark and switch off your TV or computer a couple of hours before, as they interfere with the secretion of sleep hormones.

3. One of the best ways to relieve stress and anxiety is by breathing deeply. Inhale deeply for four counts, hold it in for a moment, and then exhale for six counts. This exercise, also known as box breathing, is helpful for diffusing stress and feeling centered in your body.

4. Be grateful. Think about two or three things that you're grateful for. This may include your family, pets, freedom, music, coffee, and creativity. Anything works if it matters to you. Being grateful will expand your heart and fuel you with energy. As Tony Robbins says, you can't be grateful and fearful at the same time. Gratitude is a powerful antidote for fear, anxiety, and stress.

5. Make time to relax every day. It is important to have a relaxation routine that can help you wind down and be mellow. Some good ways to wind down include watching comedy shows, running, walking, doing yoga, and taking a relaxing bath. My favorite relaxation activities include listening to my favorite music and enjoying a one-hour body massage using lavender oil.

6. Talking and laughing with family and friends opens your heart and nurtures your spirit. It strengthens your mind and prepares you to take on life with full confidence. When you know that your friends and family have got your back, it makes you happy and resilient.

7. Dr. Deepak Chopra recommends walking barefoot on the natural surfaces of earth. The earth has healing energy within itself, and when you touch your feet on its surface, you can access it.

What is the human spirit? The human spirit is the

incorporeal part of man. The Bible says that the human spirit is the breath of Almighty God and was breathed into man at the beginning of God's creation. It is the human spirit that gives us a consciousness of self and other remarkable, though limited, "God-like" qualities. The human spirit includes our intellect, emotions, fears, passions, and creativity. It is this spirit that provides us the unique ability to comprehend, understand and empathize with others.

Can prayer and meditation reduce aging and extend your life? Scientific evidence suggests regular meditation can improve psychological conditions like anxiety and depression, which can affect mortality in turn. Meditation has been proven to bolster the immune system and reduce levels of cortisol, known as the stress hormone. Elevated levels of cortisol are linked to higher mortality through heart-related conditions, such as atherosclerosis and metabolic syndrome.

A review of two randomized controlled trials was published in *The American Journal of Cardiology* and were aimed at examining the effects of meditation specifically on mortality. The first group included participants with mild hypertension (high blood pressure) who lived in an elderly residence with an average age of eighty-one years; the second group included community-dwelling older adults with an average age of sixty-seven years.

Participants were split into groups and given instruction in either Transcendental Meditation, mindfulness meditation, mental relaxation, or progressive muscle relaxation techniques. The control group participants were offered general health education classes. Transcendental Meditation is described as a simple technique that involves sitting comfortably with the eyes closed for fifteen to twenty minutes per session, twice a day, to achieve a state of "restful alertness." Mindfulness meditation training focuses on breathing and observing thoughts dispassionately as they arise in the mind. Study subjects using mental relaxation techniques were encouraged to repeat a phrase or verse to themselves during each session. Finally, subjects using progressive muscle relaxation were coached to gradually let go of tension in each major muscle group to promote an overall state of calm.

Participants were evaluated after three months. The Transcendental Meditation groups from both trials reported significantly lower blood pressure than the other meditation and control groups, but it's the long-term data that is most fascinating. The researchers followed up on the original trials to determine the vital status of the participants, which was obtained from the National Death Index maintained by the National Center for Health Statistics. Of the 202 subjects in the original two clinical trials, 101 had died on follow-up. These mortalities were coded based on the International Classification of Diseases (ICD-9) to determine the cause of death. The results revealed that after an average of 7.6 years (up to a maximum of almost nineteen years), the subjects practicing transcendental meditation were 23 percent less likely to die of any cause during that period and 30 percent less likely to die of cardiovascular disease during the same period. Subjects were also 49 percent less likely to die of cancer during the follow-up period.

The authors of the review – Robert Schneider, MD; Charles Alexander; Frank Staggers, MD; Stephen Arndt, PhD; Vernon Barnes, PhD; and Stanford Nidich, Edh – suggest that the benefits of meditation are almost as good as those resulting from drug therapy for hypertension, without the side effects, though they do not recommend using meditation instead of medication proved to lower high blood pressure. According to the authors, this is the first long-term analysis of the effect of non-drug therapies on the mortality rate for people with elevated blood pressure. Two important questions remain: Will meditation improve longevity for people with normal blood pressure? And which type of relaxation or meditation technique provides the greatest longevity benefit? Though future research might answer these questions with greater certainty, many are happily satisfied with the boosts of energy and well-being that meditation offers in the short-term. Get started and try to incorporate a regular meditation practice into your life.

In their book *Life Force*, Tony Robbins; Peter Diamandis, MD; and Robert Hariri, MD, PhD, provide us with a checklist to reduce aging and to enjoy health, fitness, and longevity.

1. Hydrate. Drink half your weight in ounces of water per day. Add some fresh lemon and a pinch of Celtic sea salt to optimize your hydration and electrolyte balance.
2. Eat food closest to their natural source. Avoid processed carbs and low-quality processed meats.
3. Decrease disease risk. Consume at least one serving of vegetables per day, including broccoli, sprouts, cauliflower, or kale.
4. Commit to a structured eating time frame. Consume meals for an eight to twelve hours and fast for a twelve- to sixteen-hour window each day.
5. Stay consistent with sleep. Go to sleep and wake up about the same time each day.
6. Get strong. Perform three resistance training sessions per week.
7. Strengthen your heart, lungs, and build endurance with three cardiovascular exercise sessions of twenty to thirty minutes each session.
8. Consider the power of using the heat and cold to use positive stressors to lower your blood pressure, reduce inflammation, reduce your risk of Alzheimer's, and cut your risk of cardiovascular disease by 50 percent.
9. Train your brain with daily breathwork and meditation for five-twenty minutes per day.

In summary, aging is not a disease. Longevity health practices must begin in early life, including taking care of your immune system, relieving stress and anxiety, and nourishing a healthy brain.

9

SENIOR HOUSING, AND LIVING WITH COMPASSION AND AWARENESS

"To care for those who once cared for us is one of the highest honors."
— Tia Walker

Not that long ago, there were basically two options for senior living: living independently in one's own home or apartment or full-time skilled nursing care. The assisted living concept was created to provide an additional option bridging the two. To help you find senior housing that suits your needs or the needs of your loved ones, here are some options for your consideration.

Assisted living is a community-based, long-term living arrangement designed for seniors who need some help with the activities of daily living but who want to preserve as much independence as possible. Typically, the help seniors get in assisted living facilities is individualized to meet each resident's needs and desires. Depending on the situation, services can be added or removed as circumstances and choices dictate.

No single description can paint a complete picture of what assisted living is. One community may look like a modern high-rise apartment building. Another might look like a quiet suburban townhome community. Still another may resemble a resort hotel or a country club. But we can make some generalizations. Seniors who live in assisted living communities typically will have their own private, apartment-style living quarters, with convenient shared services on site and nearby. Services usually include meals, social and recreational activities, and varying levels of therapeutic and medical assistance. Another generalization: Residents of assisted living communities are overwhelmingly satisfied with those communities and the lifestyles they afford.

There is no single national standard that defines what assisted living communities must provide. Providers are licensed at the state level, so the requirements of what it takes to offer assisted living services vary from state to state. Just as you would with any product or service you buy, ask any provider you are considering what is included with the basic monthly fees and what services are available at extra cost. It's also a good idea to check with your state's licensing authority to learn what are your state's standards.

You might hear the term "continuum of care" associated with the assisted living concept. Some senior-focused communities say that they offer the complete continuum of care, from independent living to twenty-four-hour skilled nursing care. If independent living is at one end of the continuum and full-time skilled nursing care at the other, you might deduce – correctly – that assisted living is in between the two. It is a "happy medium," if you will.

If you ask seniors in the United States what is most important to them, maintaining as much independence as possible is a nearly universal answer. As we age, we might remain largely healthy and vigorous, yet still find one or more of the activities of daily living increasingly difficult to manage on our own. Sometimes a spouse, family member, or friend can help us. But if not, should skilled nursing care be the only alternative? In hindsight, it seems obvious it should not. Yet before assisted living was developed, those were basically the options.

You will hear the term "continuum of care" used most often in the context of senior living communities that include separate but adjacent sections offering independent living, assisted living, and twenty-four-hour skilled nursing care. These appeal to seniors and their loved ones who know that the senior adult can remain within one community setting and maintain the optimal balance of independence and assistance as time goes on.

The cost of assisted living is typically billed monthly. Many communities offer tiered pricing so that residents who need or want fewer services can pay less, with costs increasing as more services are included. Those who are now living independently but exploring assisted living as a potential option for the future often find that the cost seems high. But they usually are not making an apples-to-apples comparison. Far from being "just an apartment," assisted living includes many living expenses you might take for granted. Daily meals are usually one of those expenses. Many people vastly underestimate their monthly costs for food. Not only are residents of assisted living communities sparing the expense of buying food for their meals, but they are also spared the time and effort of shopping for and cooking all of their meals.

Utilities, such as electricity, water, and gas service, are also typically included, as are maintenance of the grounds and the living quarters themselves. Then, too, there are some benefits of assisted living whose costs are difficult to quantify, such as greater measures of safety, security, and community. While it's true that costs among different communities themselves can vary widely, when comparing the cost to independent living, be sure to take all that is included into account.

We can, however, make some generalizations about costs. According to Genworth's 2016 Cost of Care Survey, the median average cost for assisted living in the US is $3,628 per month, or $43,539 annually. (Actual quotes may differ from what is presented based on timing and services required.) The level of services provided and other factors can cause the costs of communities in the same area to vary widely. Cost will also vary by region. Where the general cost of living is higher, the cost of assisted living will most likely be higher as well.

Most people pay for assisted living through their financial resources. This might mean using some combination of a pension or annuity, plus savings and investments. Sometimes, financial help from one's children or other family members comes into play.

Seniors who own the home they live in might see that asset as an ideal way to finance the cost. They may, for instance, choose to sell their home outright and use the proceeds to pay for assisted living. Or they may rent the home. A third option is a reverse mortgage, which allows one to borrow against the equity of the home while retaining ownership of it. If you decide to use your home or another real estate you own to finance your care costs, be sure you understand all of the details and ramifications of such an arrangement.

For many, long-term care insurance offers a good way to finance a comfortable lifestyle at the facility of their choice. Do your homework, though, because several factors can affect your long-term care insurance costs and benefits. Some government programs, such as veterans' or Medicaid benefits, may help pay for care, though that help may be somewhat limited. Medicaid policies vary greatly from state to state.

Few people factor senior living care into their long-term financial planning. While there are understandable reasons for this, the more you plan, the more options you will have should the need arise. Still, chances are there are assisted living communities near you that will meet the needs and budget of you or your loved ones. The services offered by assisted living providers will vary depending on the community. Some communities offer services in a range of tiers and fees, so the services you receive can be customized to your needs. In general, basic services provided will include comfortable private living quarters, twenty-four-hour security and supervision, emergency call systems in each apartment, daily meals and snacks, housekeeping and laundry service, medication services, wellness and fitness programs, social and recreational activities, and shopping and transportation assistance.

In a Nursing Home report by written by Claire Simmons, over 1.4 million people in the United States currently receive long-term care in a nursing home. This number is expected to double by the year 2050. Unfortunately, with over 15,700 nursing homes in the country, the quality of care provided in each nursing home can vary substantially. This is a major concern for families and residents. How do they know the facility is reputable and safe and has a caring staff? Seniors are one of the country's most vulnerable populations. Often, ensuring the safety and security of the nursing home facility is a duty that falls to the senior's family, usually their adult children. Nursing home facilities are subject to strict regulation and oversight. They are often regulated on the state, (by state health departments) and city levels or by local regulations and ordinances. Nursing home facilities are also regulated on the federal level. This is because nursing home facilities are funded by federal Medicaid funds.

To understand how nursing homes are regulated, the basic functions of the facility must first be established. Nursing homes throughout the United States provide twenty-four-hour skilled medical care for seniors. Typically, the senior will require at least some degree of assistance with one or more activities required for daily living. Activities which require assistance include dressing, preparing meals, bathing, and other hygiene-related issues. Management of prescription medication and other medical care is another major service provided by nursing home facilities. Over half of all nursing home residents are over the age of eighty-five. This age group is expected to increase until the year 2026. Additionally, the Centers for Disease Control and Prevention expects that more than 2.8 million people will need nursing home care by 2050. As the nursing home population grows, proper oversight will be necessary to ensure both existing and new facilities are safe, accountable, and secure.

On March 25, 2016, the *Nursing Home Data Compendium for 2015* was published. This document, created by the Department of Health and Human Services, pulled data from three major sources: the Community Assessment for Public Health Emergency Response (CASPER) database for survey and certification information, the U.S. Census Bureau for population data, and the Minimum Data Set (MDS). CASPER is designed to provide public health leaders and emergency managers information about a community so they can make informed decisions. The U.S. Census Bureau is the leading source of statistical information about the nation's people. Our population statistics come from decennial censuses, which count the entire U.S. population every ten years, along with several other surveys. The Minimum Data Set is part of a federally mandated process for clinical assessment of all residents in Medicare or Medicaid certified nursing homes. This process entails a comprehensive, standardized assessment of each resident's functional capabilities and health needs. Assessments are conducted by trained nursing home clinicians on all patients at admission and discharge, in addition to other time intervals (e.g., quarterly, annually, and when residents experience a significant change in status).

Overall, the results were generally positive and reassuring. The number of deficiency-free facilities increased from 8.8 percent in 2009 to 10.2 percent in 2005. Note, this is an increase in facilities that were found to be free from issues. This is a reversal of a previous downward trend. From 2005 to 2008, reports of health deficiencies in nursing facilities were on the increase. Regulation and other factors have helped decrease health deficiencies. There are five major categories of health deficiencies.

1.   Improper storage and/ or cooking of food

2. Accidents caused to residents due, at least in part, to lack of employee supervision
3. Accidents caused to residents due, at least in part, to improperly maintained facilities
4. Improper resident care involving physical and mental wellbeing
5. Lack of proper measures to control and prevent the spread of infections

Some of these are also considered deficiencies in the quality of care. The good news is findings of substandard care have also decreased. In 2008, substandard care reports were at 4.4 percent. This dropped to 3.2 percent in 2014. The report also identified states with an increase in nursing homes as well as ones with a decrease. Nineteen states had an increase in the number of facilities. Of those, the biggest increases were in Alaska (20 percent increase), Nevada (8.2 percent increase), and Arizona (5.8 percent increase). States with the biggest decline in facilities were Vermont (7.5 percent decline), North Dakota (5.9 percent decline), and Maine (4.6 percent decline).

Selecting a quality nursing home is often a job for the adult child of the senior who is looking for nursing home care. Unfortunately, there is no real shortcut here. Finding a high-quality nursing home requires time and legwork. Experts recommend a visit to the nursing home. While a scheduled visit is usually a great step initially, searchers are encouraged to stop by the facility during the day unannounced. This will help determine both a more accurate picture of day-to-day activities as well as general security of the facility.

There are two major areas that can reveal a lot about the state of the entire nursing home: the facility and the staff. An older facility is not necessarily inferior, while a newer facility isn't necessarily superior. The important issue is the current state of the facility. First, is the facility clean? Next, is it well-maintained? Even a high-quality nursing home will have ongoing maintenance issues. The issue is how quickly and efficiently maintenance issues are handled. Additionally, nursing home maintenance requires special challenges. Nursing homes require a calm, quiet atmosphere. Is any construction kept away from the residents as much as possible? Are the maintenance employees friendly and eager to interact with the residents? Does the staff treat the residents with friendliness and respect? Obviously, even the worst staff will be on their best behavior during the initial meeting. Therefore, experts recommend unscheduled visits. Also, established residents are often another useful source of information.

Aside from the courteous professionalism, staff availability is another major factor in overall resident safety. The staff-to-resident ratio should be high enough to ensure residents are never left unattended or in potentially dangerous situations. The Nursing Home Data Compendium brought a lot of relief to anyone looking for nursing home care. Substandard quality of care and health deficiency are at an eleven-year low. As the population ages and nursing home care is required by more and more people, the recent report adds a bit of reassurance to anyone hesitant about finding a quality facility.

Independent living, often referred to as retirement living, is the term applied to a senior lifestyle that maintains an active nature and level of independence. Where many seniors could use the valuable extra assistance that comes with home care or assisted living, others don't require that level of care and seek a more active lifestyle and community. Independent living and retirement communities help seniors achieve this by providing an environment where retired adults can live among their peers while taking advantage of the many amenities and activities these communities provide. Picking the right retirement community for you is a big choice. Search the independent living communities close to where you want to live and read reviews to see what other seniors and their families have to say about their experiences. According to SeniorAdvisor.com, the average consumer rating for independent living communities on SeniorAdvisor.com is four stars out of five. Independent living communities in Nebraska, Rhode Island, and Kansas tend to be rated higher than the national average, whereas communities in Mississippi, New Jersey, and Delaware tend to be rated lower. The states with the most independent living communities are California, Texas, and Florida.

How much does independent living cost? As for amenities, living quarters, and property values vary for different independent living communities, there's a wide range in community costs.

In general, most retirement villages or communities average $3,500 a month. Actual quotes may differ from what is presented based on timing and services required. Often, that includes features like regular meals, healthcare on staff, and access to fitness facilities and other amenities on site. When it comes to independent living options, communities offer an array of features and amenities. Not every item listed below is available at every retirement community, but this list gives you some idea of what to expect and look for. Some of the common services you can expect to find are a variety of activities offered onsite; ranging from movie nights; knitting groups; educational classes; trips to nearby sites; meals offered by the independent community's onsite chef; fitness options, such as work out equipment, pools, or hiking trails; senior apartments (many with features like kitchens or balconies); senior houses; transportation services; medical staff onsite (or that come for visits); and even beauty and hair services.

Memory care is specialized care provided to those with varying degrees of dementia or Alzheimer's disease. It involves creating a safe, structured, home-like environment that enables residents to enjoy as fulfilling a life as possible. Alzheimer's disease is typically referred to in three stages: early, middle, and late stage.

Many people are familiar with the early (or mild) and the late (or severe) stages but not sure what to expect from the middle stage. Moderate, or middle stage, Alzheimer's is generally the longest stage of the disease, with some living in the stage for several years. As the disease progresses, family members and caregivers may notice behaviors such as needing assistance performing daily tasks, such as bathing or dressing; difficulty following a conversation or remembering details about what day it is or their family history; withdrawal from social situations; behavior or more frequent mood changes, including becoming agitated; suspicion of others; changes in sleep patterns, such as wanting to sleep more during the day; and difficulty sleeping at night.

Medicine's understanding of Alzheimer's and its effects on the human brain is still in the pioneering phases. While we learn more all the time about how genetics, life events, and lifestyle components are involved in catalyzing the initial signs and progression of Alzheimer's, the cure remains elusive. The more you remain up to date on the current research and studies' findings, including Alzheimer's facts, figures, and stats, the better you can improve the quality of life for yourself and the ones you love. The following facts are derived from two helpful Alzheimer's disease resources: The NIH's page on Alzheimer's Disease Facts and Alzinfo.org.

- AD is the sixth-leading cause of death in the United States.
- Most people with late-onset AD exhibit signs and symptoms as early as their sixties, even if the diagnosis doesn't happen until much later.
- Experts believe that AD-related changes in the brain may start as much as ten years before the beginning symptoms are detectable.
- Early-onset AD comprises about 10 percent of the Alzheimer's population and is typically noticed/ diagnosed between the ages of thirty and sixty.
- Someone is diagnosed with AD about every sixty-five seconds.

- Doctors predict as many as fourteen million Americans will be living with Alzheimer's by the year 2050.
- One-third of all seniors die with Alzheimer's or some other dementia-related condition
- It costs about $350,000 per person to support the long-term health and wellbeing of an AD patient.
- There are multiple forms of AD and dementia – early-onset, late-onset, Parkinson's-related, et cetera. Care and treatment plans may vary depending on the type.
- Alzheimer's genes are identified, but they are not the sole cause of AD, nor does the presence of the genes mean an individual will get AD.

There is no specific treatment for AD or dementia, although some slow its progression. Certain lifestyle changes have been shown to slow down the progression of AD. These last two points are part of what makes living with Alzheimer's so challenging. Currently, there are not always clear reasons why a person has the disease, and there is no tried-and-true treatment for AD. Recent studies have shown that high-fat, high-sugar diets "prime the brain" for AD. Diets that are higher in fats, sugars, and processed foods contribute to inflammation in both the hippocampus and the frontal lobe of the brain, two areas that experience AD decline.

In closing this chapter, if you or your loved ones need the services of any of these long-term living arrangements, especially memory care, I recommend that you make the necessary legal arrangements if something happens to you. Ensuring the property, if any is transferred to the right party when the time comes is a key aspect of estate planning. A life estate and an irrevocable trust are two different methods to go about this, each with its own advantages and disadvantages. I highly recommend the creation of a living will or trust on file with an attorney or a trusted family member. A living will informs your doctors about your preferences for medical care at the end of life. There are five main types of trusts: living trust, testamentary trust, revocable trust, an irrevocable trust, and funded or unfunded trust. Each different kind has its own uses and purposes and because these are legal documents, you should use an estate planning attorney to help you understand, write, and execute them.

10

BONUS CHAPTER ON ADOPTING TECHNOLOGIES AND ADVANCING RESEARCH

"Technology like art is a soaring exercise of the human imagination."
— Daniel Bell

This is a bonus chapter designed to provide you with information about effective public health measures to support your healthy longevity. Maybe you've heard of the term "biohacking." It's the use of technology or supplements to create effective shortcuts to achieve a result. Depending on your physical, mental, and emotional condition, you may want to consider using some of the following technologies or supplements to improve your biological age.

I enjoyed learning about my biological age by taking a blood test to reveal my true age. If you're wondering whether your healthy (or unhealthy) lifestyle is having an impact, then you've probably heard about your biological age – that is, how your body is aging compared to average rather than just how many years you have lived in it (called your chronological age). There are several ways to measure your biological age, each with its own pros and cons, but one of the most popular and accurate is looking at how your DNA structure is fairing with age, which is called epigenetic age.

Are you wondering what is epigenetics and how is it

different from genetics? "Epi" is a Greek prefix for "above." Genetics is the study of our DNA. Together, epigenetics means the study of things above and beyond the genome. This means we are studying the changes to your DNA and how it affects the body instead of what the DNA could possibly do or mean. It is often more useful than genetics because it allows us to see how the genetic material in your body behaves instead of just seeing what it contains.

As we age, we have changes other than what happens epigenetically to our DNA. One of the biggest changes to our health and bodies is called immunosenescence. Immunosenescence is when our immune systems become weaker and less functional as we age. This is often seen in the blood by having a fewer number of naive T-cells and a higher number of senescent T-cells. There are other changes in the number and percentage of cells that make up the blood as well. And because of these changes, we see health consequences like older individuals being more likely to die from the flu or COVID-19.

Traditional genetics is like looking at a light bulb and its components but not knowing if the bulb is producing light. Epigenetics lets us know if the light bulb is on or off. Well, I am happy to report that my light bulb in on. The link between epigenetics and health has been linked through biological age. This is important because aging is the leading risk factor for multiple chronic diseases and disorders. Therefore, finding a way to slow the biological aging process is essential. Our epigenetic clock is the most accurate measurement of biological age and age-related disease risk. Epigenetic aging can be reversed, so it is crucial to understand DNA methylation changes through utilizing TruAge™. Since we know that aging can be reversed, we can apply changes to our lifestyles and use TruAge™ to show that we are reducing our risk of incidence of disease and death.

Race seems to have a significant impact on epigenetics. We are unsure now how much this affects different health outcomes, but studies have shown the following:

- Infants from mixed race/ ethnicity origin had significantly higher methylation age and higher frequency of fast aging rate than that in African-origin Black people.
- African Americans have indications of a significantly younger immune system age than Caucasians after controlling for gender, educational level, diabetes status, and Hypertension.
- According to measures of extrinsic epigenetic age acceleration, Hispanics have a significantly older extrinsic epigenetic age than Caucasians and fewer naïve CD4+ T cells. The T helper cells (T h cells), also known as CD4 + cells or CD4-positive cells, are a type of T cell that play an important role in the immune system.
- In one famous study, there were three variables linked to extrinsic epigenetic age acceleration: race/ ethnicity, hypertension, and gender. However, this significant association between extrinsic epigenetic age acceleration and hypertension, type 2 diabetes status is only found in Caucasians, not in African Americans.
- The lower level of intrinsic epigenetic age acceleration in Hispanics echoes the finding that Hispanics in the US have a lower overall risk of mortality than Caucasians, despite having a disadvantaged risk profile. The fact that Hispanics have typically had lower intrinsic epigenetic aging, but not lower extrinsic epigenetic aging might reflect that Hispanics have higher levels of metabolic/ inflammatory risk profiles and have a lower relative CD4+ T cell percentage than Caucasians.
- Sex morbidity-mortality paradox refers to the observation that women have a lower mortality rate compared to men despite being more likely to suffer from other diseases and co-morbid conditions. It has always been assumed that this might be due

to behavioral traits, such as lifestyle factors, or that they might be less likely to go to a doctor to be diagnosed with a disease or condition.

Often, knowing how to be the healthiest you can be is difficult. My primary doctor has measured all kinds of tests including blood levels like cholesterol, inflammation, and blood sugar. She has performed tests such as colonoscopies, vision tests, and physical function tests. Now, with this TruAge™ single measurement, I can link my health and longevity to a single, simple test that can help me and my doctor know the best way to address my health concerns in a personalized way. I am happy to report that based on my TruAge™ test, my true biological age is fifty-nine versus my chronological age of seventy-two years old. I guess I must be doing something right. For more information, visit https://trudiagnostic.com/.

I am also enjoying Bits® plant-based nutrition tablets made purely of algae, such as Spirulina (an energizing and nourishing algae) and Chlorella (a health and wellness algae), which support your body naturally.

Spirulina – blue-green algae grown in some of the most beautiful places in the world – has been well-researched for its many potential benefits. Some of the most significant health benefits include detoxing heavy metals, eliminating candida, fighting cancer, and lowering blood pressure. Each serving contains a good amount of spirulina protein plus important vitamins and minerals like copper, iron, riboflavin and thiamine. This algae has a rich history. Although there are several distinct differences between chlorella and spirulina, the two are often confused. Spirulina may cause autoimmune reactions in some who are susceptible to autoimmunity. It's also not recommended for pregnant women or children. Be cautious where you purchase Spirulina, as it may be contaminated if not bought from a high-quality source, leading to additional spirulina side effects.

People use Chlorella for many different health concerns. Here are seven scientifically proven chlorella benefits you can hope to receive by incorporating this superfood into your daily diet.

Chlorella detoxifies heavy metals. If you have mercury fillings in your teeth, eat fish regularly, have been exposed to radiation, or consume foods from China, you may have heavy metals lurking in your body. It is important for your overall health and wellness to be proactive in detoxing heavy metals and toxins.

Chlorella detoxifies radiation and chemotherapy. Radiation therapy and chemotherapy are the most common forms of cancer treatment today. Anyone who has gone through either of these treatments or knows anyone who has knows what a toll they take on the body. Chlorella's high levels of chlorophyll have been shown to protect the body against ultraviolet radiation treatments while removing radioactive particles from the body.

Chlorella supports your immune system. Research published in 2012 in the *Nutrition Journal* found that after eight weeks of chlorella intake, natural killer cell activity improved. Researchers from the Yonsei University in Seoul Korea studied healthy individuals and their immune system's response to chlorella supplements.

Chlorella promotes weight loss. Losing weight is difficult, especially as we age. In a study published in the Journal of Medicinal Food, researchers state, "Chlorella intake resulted in noticeable reductions in body fat percentage, serum total cholesterol, and fasting blood glucose levels." Chlorella benefits you by helping to regulate hormones, helping with metabolism, improving circulation, and promoting higher levels of energy. It also helps to reduce weight and body fat and removes stored toxins. As our bodies lose weight, toxins are released and can be reabsorbed. It is important to flush these toxins out of our system as quickly as possible. Chlorella's ability to surround the toxins and heavy metals resident in our bodies helps facilitate elimination and prevent reabsorption. For more information about Bits®, visit https://www.energybits.com/

The following are new technologies and advanced research that you can investigate and apply to your medical needs. Have fun researching the following companies and their offerings.

Docere Clinics provide the highest-quality, most comprehensive stem cell procedure available in the world, delivered with complete integrity and human compassion. For more information, visit https://www.docereclinics.com.

The BioCharger NG is a hybrid subtle energy revitalization platform. The transmitted energy stimulates and invigorates the entire body to optimize and improve potential health, wellness, and athletic performance. For more information, visit https://biocharger.com.

Adaptive resistance exercise with ARX provides you with the most effective workout in as little as ten minutes a week. Short for Adaptive Resistance Exercise, ARX is scientifically proven to deliver quantifiable results in less time. For more information, visit https://quantifyfitness.com/what-is-adaptive-resistance.

The Ballancer®Pro is the safest and most state-of-the-art compression therapy system. Backed by decades of medical research and based on the principles of manual lymphatic drainage this FDA-cleared technology is "light years" ahead of any compression therapy system. For more information, visit https://ballancerpro.com.

Regenerative Medicine provides advanced hair treatments by Alan J. Bauman, MD, ABHRS, IAHRS, FISHRS, a full-time hair transplant surgeon who founded a medical practice, Bauman Medical, in Boca Raton, Florida, in 1997 and has treated nearly 30,000 patients and performed over 10,000 hair transplant procedures to date. For more information, visit https://www.baumanmedical.com.

Beam Minerals was founded by Dan Howard and Caroline Alan as a vehicle for promoting the amazing power of plant-based fulvic and humic minerals. For more information, visit https://www.beamminerals.com.

BiOptimizers help you shift into peak biologically

optimized health, an optimal state of well-being in the body, mind, and soul. BiOptimizers will help you to build more muscle and lose fat and improve athletic performance. For more information visit https://bioptimizers.com.

Sleepme is a product you need to check out if you are not enjoying a good night's sleep. For more information, visit https://sleep.me.

Essentia is an organic mattress independently named by internationally renowned wellness institutes. Essentia is packed with non-toxic certified organic vegan technology. For more information, visit https://myessentia.com.

Eng3's patented NanoVi® technology produces the same biological signal your body makes to repair cell damage brought on by free radicals (also known as reactive oxygen species or ROS). For more information, visit https://eng3corp.com.

H-Wave is a multi-functional electrical stimulation device intended to speed recovery, restore function, and manage chronic, acute, or post-operative pain. It is a non-invasive, drug-free, alternative treatment option without harmful side effects. For more information visit https://www.h-wave.com.

HOCATT helps harmonize multiple modalities into the ultimate wellness symphony. Combining ten highly effective technologies, perfectly sequenced to activate one another, it provides integrated support for promotion of maximum health and wellness. For more information, visit https://hocatt.com/hct-pro.

Hyperbaric oxygen therapy (HBOT) is the medical use of oxygen in a pressurized environment, at a level higher than one atmosphere absolute (ATA). Increased pressure allows for oxygen to dissolve and saturate the blood plasma (independent of hemoglobin/red blood cells), which yields a broad variety of positive physiological, biochemical, and cellular effects. For more information, visit https://www.oxyhealth.com.

Power Plate's patented PrecisionWave™ technology is

engineered to activate the body's natural reflexive response to precision vibration, engaging the muscles in a consistent and controlled manner that results in accelerated training benefits. For more information, visit https://powerplate.com.

Pure Wave is a powerful massage tool that allows you to create a completely personalized massage experience. The patented dual-mode GEN II adjusts to your needs wherever you are in your self-healing journey. For more information, visit https://www.padousa.com.

Sunlighten infrared saunas can help reduce wrinkles and crow's feet while improving overall skin tone, softness, smoothness, elasticity, clarity, and firmness. For more information, visit https://www.sunlighten.com.

TrueDark's premium blue light glasses help you manage artificial light (a.k.a. junk light) exposure so you can work smarter, sleep deeper, and feel your best. For more information, visit https://truedark.com.

TrueLight is a wellness technology brand that is committed to improving health and performance using light. The use of patent pending innovative red-light therapy devices helps you look, feel and perform better. For more information, visit https://shoptruelight.com.

Alpha-Stim electrotherapy device is proven effective and safe for pain management and treatment of anxiety, insomnia, and depression. It helps you fight both the sleepless nights and the overwhelming sadness that can make it hard to get out of bed in the morning. For more information, visit https://www.alpha-stim.com.

InBody devices are non-invasive and convenient, making them the ideal tool to implement into nutrition programs for body composition analysis. The InBody test provides comprehensive results that can be used to track and educate clients on body fat and health risk as well as understand the differences in diet consumption effects. For more information, visit https://inbodyusa.com.

Plunging into cold water triggers the production of the

neurotransmitter norepinephrine, a critical chemical in the body that helps regulate attention, focus, and energy. A daily cold plunge can help increase your levels of norepinephrine, simultaneously increasing your energy. For more information, visit https://thecoldplunge.com.

WAVi's Medical Platform provides a multifaceted tool for practitioners to measure brain performance. The WAVi Medical Platform includes the measurement of brain wave patterns. For more information, visit https://wavimed.com.

It is interesting to note that currently, in the United States, aging is not considered a medical condition. As far as the medical advance research is concerned, I am encouraged by all the research on aging that is being done at Harvard University, my alma mater. You may also want to follow the research work being performed by Dr. David Sinclair, Dr. Marc Lipsitch and Dr. George Church at the Harvard Medical School. Marc Lipsitch, is an American epidemiologist and professor in the Department of Epidemiology at the Harvard T.H. Chan School of Public Health, where he is the director of the Center for Communicable Disease Dynamics. And George McDonald Church is an American geneticist, molecular engineer, and chemist. He is the Robert Winthrop Professor of Genetics at Harvard Medical School, professor of health sciences and technology at Harvard and MIT, and a founding member of the Wyss Institute for Biologically Inspired Engineering. David Andrew Sinclair is a professor of genetics and co-director of the Paul F. Glenn Center for Biology of Aging Research at Harvard Medical School. He is known for his research on aging with a focus on epigenetics. In a recent book, *Lifespan*, written by Dr. Sinclair and Dr. Matthew D. La Plate, they shared with us the amazing global effort to stop aging and the likely possibility of a future where aging can be treated like any other disease.

In summary, I am optimistic about their gene therapy and research work of these world's foremost medical experts on aging and genetics and their groundbreaking new theory that will forever change the way we think about why we age and what we can do about it. I, for one, intend to expand my life for another forty years and to slow down or even reverse my genetic clock by applying emerging technologies and simple lifestyle changes, such as intermittent fasting, cold exposures, and exercising, which are shown to lead to longer lives.

11

RESIGNATION TO DYING YOUNG

*"Resignation is what kills people. Once they've rejected resignation,
humans gain the privilege of making humanity their footpath."*
— Kouta Hirano

Throughout this book, I have shared ideas about ways to extend your lifetime horizon. Yet I know that some of you, even after agreeing with these ideas, will not implement them for many reasons, including lack of self-love. Yes, lack of self-love – nothing else will explain you not taking action to make the necessary changes to extend your lifetime horizon. Is it so hard to have fun, laugh, enjoy music, eat well, and enjoy your stress-free life?

Some of you will decide to continue to eat incorrectly because you will feel that you are depriving yourself of the foods that you want. I know lifestyle changes are difficult to accomplish but possible if your why is big enough. Think again: Why do you want to extend your life? I know that losing weight can be beneficial for people who are overweight or obese. But why is a healthy weight important? Let me remind you that losing weight lowers the risk of type 2 diabetes, heart disease, high blood pressure, and some types of cancer.

Creating healthy habits, instead of jumping from one diet to another, is a better way to shed pounds and live a healthier lifestyle. Consider adopting these new technologies to help you in your longevity journey. If you are thinking you do not know the benefits of these new technologies, investigate and find out if you and your body can benefit from these new technologies and advance research. Maybe you consider them too expensive. Maybe so, but even more expensive will be if you end up sick and must be hospitalized. Start changing your habits by setting realistic goals. You cannot expect to change all your eating habits overnight and for the changes to last. Instead, making small changes, such as cutting out soda, can help you lose up to ten pounds in a few months. Do not make your new diet too strict and restrictive. Having a treat occasionally is delightful. Do not expect to lose the weight immediately. It took time to put it on, and it will take time for it to come off.

Do not procrastinate. Start changing your habits now. Be strong and make smart decisions with your daily food choices. Changing eating habits may cause headaches, fatigue, mental fog, confusion, and irritability. Many of this is caused by not eating enough calories or carbohydrates. Being hungry does not mean that you are losing weight. Your goal should be to find foods that make you feel fuller longer, such as fiber, protein, and good fats. Do not skip meals. This will cause you to eat even more because you will be famished. Your body needs a steady intake of glucose to increase your metabolism and feed your brain and body with energy. Crash diets rob your body of this glucose. This is unhealthy and dangerous for you. Make sure that you have adequate protein during the day, especially at lunchtime.

Do not eat dinner at least three hours before you go to bed. Remember that changes to eating habits and lifestyle changes require a lot of time. Start by planning your weekly healthy meals and dividing everything up into the right portion sizes. Take one day a week to plan your meals and to cook them and divide them up into portions. Meal planning will also save you a headache on days when you are tired from work and have no energy to cook. Instead of going for the bag of chips, you will go for that shredded chicken, which you can eat with the roasted potatoes you made last Sunday. Exercise is important for weight loss, but it should not consume all your time or money. One day a week, set up your exercise plan for the next seven days. Try to incorporate it into your daily life so that it isn't hard to keep up. Give yourself a rest day with exercise so that your body can recover. Counting calories can be one of the most frustrating and difficult things for someone to do. While it is important to decrease the number of calories that you are eating to lose weight, it is more important to be able to consume the appropriate nutrients that your body needs to work properly. Cut out empty calories. Drinking lots of water instead of soda is a great way to not only lose weight but to improve your overall health. Avoid sugar as much as possible. If you have a sweet tooth, find alternatives such as yogurt or fruit.

Always celebrate your successes. For instance, if you hit your goal to lose five pounds, treat yourself to a rejuvenating massage and/ or a spa day of beauty. Some final reasons why you may not act is because you may feel socially isolated and lonely. But I do hope that you realize the importance of having friends, developing good relationships, and being involved with interesting groups where you can do fun activities, such as reading singing, dancing, telling family stories, laughing a lot, and having fun.

In closing, I recommend that you consult with a dietician to find out what kind of lifestyle changes would be best for you based on your overall objectives.

12

CONCLUSION – LIVING HEALTHIER AND LONGER

"The secret of health for both mind and body is not to mourn for the past, not to worry about the future, or not to anticipate troubles, but to live the present moment wisely and earnestly."

— Siddartha Guatama Buddha

I have shared with you the steps that you will go through to move from feelings of despair to having the skills, tools, and resources to live a healthier, happier, and longer life.

In Chapter 4, I taught you about the importance of laughter and music in your life. Laughter is a potent releaser of endorphins. Laughing with friends releases endorphins (the chemicals that help us to feel good) in our brain via opioid receptors. Music and laughter can also bring lasting benefits to your state of mind and how therapeutic music has been clinically proven to improve sleep, relieve stress and gain more energy for your day.

In Chapter 5, I taught you about the science of fasting and longevity, a fasting-mimicking diet, and the Mediterranean diet.

In Chapter 6, I shared with you the importance of demography and diversity. What do demographics have to do with longevity, including showing you how the place you live, and your environment have an important role in your longevity?

In Chapter 7, I showed you how clean air matters for a

healthy lifestyle and the risk of air pollution and Alzheimer's risk.

In Chapter 8, I taught you about interventions to reduce aging, including how longevity must begin in early life. Also, you learned ways to naturally relieve stress and anxiety as well as the importance of volunteering and developing friends to find significance.

In Chapter 9, I shared relevant information about care-givers, including elder abuse, care managers, and families providing the right support.

In the bonus Chapter 10, I informed you about new technologies, advanced research, and digital health solu-tions, including powerful tools to increase health care qual-ity and access. I also shared with you the biology of aging versus chronological age and the dissemination of infor-mation about effective public health measures to support healthy longevity.

In Chapter 11, I reminded you of the reasons why you are unlikely to take action and what is likely to happen if they don't.

In Chapter 12, I reiterated my heartfelt desire for you to live a healthier and longer life. I, again, clarified the im-portance of having a blueprint to live healthier and longer.

I reminded you about the importance of reaching a bal-ance where people, habitat, and wildlife can coexist to min-imize air pollution; Alzheimer's risk; and how clean air mat-ters for a healthy brain. You learned about the importance of family and the caregiver's impact on longevity and how therapeutic music and laughing have been clinically proven to improve sleep, relieve stress, calm you, soothe your pet, and give you more energy for your day, impacting longevity.

According to a Tibetan proverb, the secret of living well and longer is to eat half, walk double, laugh triple, and love without measure. Also, I reminded you about the im-portance of intermittent fasting and enjoying a balance pes-catarian or Mediterranean diet. Remember that longevity must begin in early life, including taking care of your immune system, relieving stress and anxiety, and nourishing a healthy brain. We talked about ways to naturally relieve stress and anxiety as well as volunteering and developing friends to find significance. Finally, in the bonus chapter, I shared with you how you can extend your life by adopting technologies and advancing research to support healthy longevity.

Above all, keep in mind that forgiving and nurturing yourself can set the stage for better health, relationships, and general wellbeing. Self-compassion provides benefits including lower levels of anxiety and depression. Self-compassionate people recognize when they are suffering and are kind to themselves at these times, which reduces their anxiety and related depression. Positive emotions have been linked with better health, longer life, and greater wellbeing in numerous scientific studies. On the other hand, chronic anger, worry, and hostility increase the risk of developing heart disease, as people react to these feelings with raised blood pressure and stiffened blood vessels. But it isn't easy to maintain a healthy, positive emotional state. While some people come by self-compassion naturally, others must learn it.

Harvard psychologist Christopher Germer, in his book *The Mindful Path to Self-Compassion*, suggests that there are five ways to bring self-compassion into your life via physical, mental, emotional, relational, and spiritual methods. He and other experts have proposed a variety of ways to foster self-compassion. Here are a few.

1. Comfort your body. Eat something healthy. Lie down and rest your body. Massage your neck, feet, or hands. Take a walk. Do anything you can to improve how you feel physically gives you a dose of self-compassion.

2. Write a letter to yourself. Describe a situation that caused you to feel pain (a breakup with a lover, a job loss, a poorly received presentation). Write a letter

to yourself describing the situation without blaming anyone. Acknowledge your feelings.

3. Give yourself encouragement. If something bad or painful happens to you, think of what you would say to a good friend if the same thing happened to him or her. Direct these compassionate responses toward yourself.

4. Practice mindfulness. This is the nonjudgmental observation of your thoughts, feelings, and actions without trying to suppress or deny them.

In closing, I leave you with this quote from Cicero: "Enjoy the blessing of strength while you have it and do not bewail it when it is gone, unless, forsooth, you believe that youth must lament the loss of infancy, or early manhood the passing of youth. Life's racecourse is fixed; Nature has only a single path and that path is run but once, and to each stage of existence has been allotted its own appropriate quality; so that the weakness of childhood, the impetuosity of youth, the seriousness of middle life, the maturity of old age – each bear some of nature's fruit, which must be garnered in its own season."

ACKNOWLEDGMENTS

I have often heard that "when the student is ready, the teacher will appear." That was a welcome synchronicity to find my writing coach, Angela Lauria, through The Author's Way. Special thanks again to Angela Lauria, CEO and founder of The Author Incubator, for believing in me and my message. Special thanks to Madeline Kosten; my managing editor, Cory Hott; and my designer, Jennifer Stimson, for making the process seamless and easy.

Many thanks to my mentors and friends at Strategic Coach and Genius Network. And special thanks to family. My husband, Stephen, and my sons, Michael and Tommy, are my biggest fans – always have been and always will be. I love and appreciate them so much. My brothers, Francisco, Sergio, Ruben, and Eloy; and my sister, Zulema, are my proudest fans. Seeing them beam with pride over my accomplishments and having them text me encouraging thoughts means a lot to me. Thank you for your patience and for your unconditional love. Thank you for your sense of humor, your gentleness, and your acceptance. May my legacy make you proud!

To my Harvard Business School/ OPM32 friends – or, as I lovingly refer to them, The Old Guard – my gratefulness for our twenty-plus years of friendship as OPMers colleagues and friends has no bounds. We were a powerhouse team then, and we are a powerhouse team today. We are a team for life! So much love and appreciation for you all. Finally, special thanks to Gary Keller, entrepreneur, author, and founder of Keller Williams Realty International, the largest real estate company in the world. Gary's love and kindness are great role models for all business owners. I will leave you with one final thought, one of Gary's quotes: "Don't let small thinking cut your life down to size. Think big, aim high, act bold, and see just how big you can blow up your life."

ABOUT THE AUTHOR

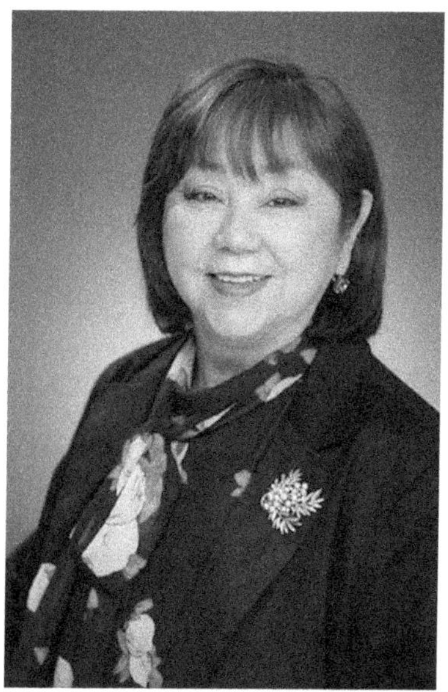

Maria Ellis, MBA, is a graduate of the Harvard Business School Owner-President Management Program and earned her bachelor's degree in business administration as well as her MBA from the University of Massachusetts in Amherst. As a former international banker, investment advisor, and financial planner, Maria has specialized in converting clients' financial objectives into successful action plans. Maria has both the know-how and the market contacts, having worked at Bank of America, Citibank, the MONY Group, Northwestern Mutual, Citi Habitats and Keller Williams.

Maria is a Chopra Certified Health Instructor, and she is the bestselling author of four books, including *Achieve Financial Freedom: The Road Map to Financial Success*; *Family Business Legacy Plan: The Ultimate Guide to Creating a Legacy for Your Family without Paying too Much in Taxes*; and *Redefining Entrepreneurial Success: A Guide to a Healthy and Holistic Lifestyle*.

Maria's background includes board leadership positions at the College of Mount Saint Vincent, the American Association of University Women, and the Virginia Gildersleeve International Fund. Maria is also a pro-bono consultant at the Harvard Business School Club of New York City Community Partners and applies her business skills to a variety of topics, including strategic planning, marketing, finance, governance, and organizational development. Maria is an active member of the Harvard Club and the Genuis Network.

THANK YOU

Thank you for reading this book! It is my great honor and pleasure to share this information with you in hopes that this book will add healthy years, even decades, to the lives of those who read it and implement healthy lifespan habits. Writing this book is, first and foremost, an act of love and gratitude; thus, I am offering you a complimentary longevity consultation. You may reach me by emailing me at mellis@fsacap.com.